PREFACE

FOR some time we have been made aware that there is a lack of a short text which reviews diet and nutrition during childhood. There are several excellent large-scale textbooks running to 300 pages and beyond and a number of books on specific nutritional topics but these are not likely to be readily available to community workers or most doctors.

Questions about diet and nutrition are among the most common which parents ask. It has also become clear that much of the advice which is given is inappropriate and is often derived from sources which lack current information. Furthermore it may often be necessary to counter beliefs derived from ill-informed media coverage. This short book is intended as a practical guide for health professionals who have no special knowledge of nutrition but who have to deal with nutritional and dietary problems and questions in children during their general work. Medical students may find it a useful introduction to the subject. We hope that it is sufficiently clearly written to be suitable reading for interested lay persons.

Its contents comprise the collective experience of a paediatrician and a paediatric dietitian who have worked together for a number of years and it aims to be a genuinely pocket-sized book. During that time, we have by discussion and sometimes by argument evolved policies for the nutritional care of ill children and for advice to the parents of healthy children. We have tried to give clear advice and policies, and not everyone will agree with all our opinions in areas where there is continued controversy. In general our policy is one of caution. In the field of diet and nutrition in children, perhaps more than in any other, Hippocrates' exhortation to first not do harm is most relevant.

We include a number of tables culled from various sources which we thought would be useful to have collected together. Wherever possible we have given the background to our views, but in a text where the essence is brevity it has not been possible, or desirable, to produce detailed argument or literature reviews. For that the reader must look elsewhere and we have appended a list of texts for possible further reading and reference.

Sheffield   L.S.T.
August 1988   B.L.W.

Handbook of Child Nutrition

L. S. TAITZ

and

B. L. WARDLEY

Department of Paediatrics
Children's Hospital, Sheffield, UK

Oxford   New York   Tokyo
OXFORD UNIVERSITY PRESS

Oxford University Press, Walton Street, Oxford OX2 6DP

Oxford New York Toronto
Delhi Bombay Calcutta Madras Karachi
Petaling Jaya Singapore Hong Kong Tokyo
Nairobi Dar es Salaam Cape Town
Melbourne Auckland

and associated companies in
Berlin Ibadan

Oxford is a trade mark of Oxford University Press

© L. S. Taitz and B. L. Wardley, 1989

First published 1989
Reprinted with corrections 1990

British Library Cataloguing in Publication Data
Taitz, Leonard S.
Handbook of child nutrition.
1. Children. Nutrition
I. Title II. Wardley, B. L. (Bridget)
613.2'088054
ISBN 0-19-261759-1
ISBN 0-19-261842-3 (pbk)

Library of Congress Cataloging in Publication Data
Taitz, Leonard S.
Handbook of child nutrition / L. S. Taitz and B. L. Wardley.
Includes index.
1. Children—Nutrition. 2. Children—Diseases—Nutritional
aspects. I. Wardley, B. (Bridget) II. Title.
RJ206.T34   1989   613.2'088054—dc19   88-37574
ISBN 0-19-261759-1
ISBN 0-19-261842-3 (pbk)

Set by Footnote Graphics, Warminster, Wilts
Printed in Great Britain by
Biddles Ltd, Guildford and Kings Lynn

CONTENTS

1

Infant feeding—
the present state of the art

THE principles for the successful feeding of the overwhelming majority of infants and children are now well understood and, although isolated problems remain, there is no reason why almost all babies and children should not be correctly fed and nourished. It is conventional and convenient to make a distinction between those infants who still depend largely on milk as their source of nutrition (sucklings) and those who eat mainly solid foods (toddlers). During the transitional intervening phase, it is convenient to describe the babies as weanlings.

FEEDING SUCKLINGS

Breast-feeding

Breast-feeding on demand remains the ideal form of feeding for young babies who are healthy, born at term, and whose parents are disposed to this form of feeding. The reasons for continuing to accept this philosophy are well set out in official statements. The needs of the young infant are constantly changing (Table 1.1). Human milk is a remarkably variable food and its changes during the period of lactation are well tailored to meet the needs of the baby during the early months of life. These first four to six months are a period of very rapid growth and development, with the brain in particular growing and developing at a rate it is not to achieve again. It is not unreasonable to suppose that the combination of amino acids and fatty acids of most breast milk and the changes which it undergoes in composition are particularly

Table 1.1 Recommended daily intakes of energy and nutrients for infants up to one year old

Age (months)	Weight (kg)	Energy (kcal[1])	Protein[3] (g[1])	Vitamins						Minerals	
				Thiamin (mg)	Riboflavin (mg)	Nicotinic acid (mg equiv.)	C (mg)	A (mg[2])	D[3] (mg)	Calcium (mg)	Iron (mg)
0–3	4.6	120	2.2	0.3	0.4	5	15	450	10	600	6
3–6	6.6	115	2.2	0.3	0.4	5	15	450	10	600	6
6–9	8.3	110	2.0	0.3	0.4	5	15	450	10	600	6
9–12	9.5	105	2.0	0.3	0.4	5	15	450	10	600	6

[1] Per kg body weight.
[2] Retinol equivalent.
[3] Cholecalciferol.

(Adapted from: DHSS 1985, Recommended Daily amounts of Food Energy and Nutrients for groups of People in the United Kingdom. Report NO15 HMSO, London)

well suited to meet these needs. This does not mean that the composition of fat and protein in breast milk is necessarily constant since the content of essential amino acids and fatty acids are by their nature determined by the content in the mother's diet.

Suckling a baby at the breast can have important emotional effects on the relationship of mother to child. It seems likely that attachment of the mother to her baby is assisted by the close physical contact and also by the pleasure which successful breast-feeding evokes.

Breast milk is probably satisfactory for larger preterm infants, but some uncertainty surrounds its use in the tinier, very preterm infants. There are few absolute contra-indications to breast-feeding. These include galactosaemia, alactasia (hereditary absence of the gut enzyme lactase), and certain drugs that the mother may have to take during the lactation period and which cross into breast milk.

Most mothers who genuinely wish to breast-feed their babies are able to overcome minor problems, with suitable support, and should succeed. Of the mothers who leave hospital breast-feeding, about two-thirds are still doing so six weeks later but by four months this has fallen to only 26 per cent. Many of those who give up were not fully committed to breast-feeding in the first place and were induced to try by the general climate favouring the method in the antenatal clinics. The most important factor which determines the prevalence of breast-feeding is parental motivation. This seems more a matter for health education and the further advance of a general climate of opinion than for specific intervention by health workers. Breast-feeding remains a social-class-determined phenomenon, heavily slanted towards the most educated section of the community. It is particularly disturbing that the rate of breast-feeding appears to have fallen recently among single-parent mothers and those having their first baby. Mothers who do not breast-feed their firstborns are very unlikely to breast-feed subsequent infants.

Some mothers are not successful in breast-feeding their babies despite wishing to do so. There are many reasons for this. As we have noted, in some mothers the commitment to breast-feed is not strong and any untoward event leads to abandonment. Breast-feeding is not an entirely instinctive process, and mothers, particularly those breast-feeding for the first time, require a great deal of help, support, and encouragement during the early stages. As the vast majority of babies are now born in hospital, it is here that this process must begin, with encouragement of demand feeding and avoiding the provision of supplementary feeds or drinks of dextrose water.

Continued support at home is also necessary. This is initially provided by the midwife and later by the health visitor. This dual system of care is desirable for several reasons but does have the potential for confused advice or crossed signals. Midwives and health visitors should communicate with each other and ensure that they share a common philosophy. Mothers will often say that they have received contradictory advice and information. This is quite frequently a cause of difficulty, particularly if the mother is also being given advice by general practitioners, community doctors, or paediatricians. This conflict may arise from genuine differences of opinion, hence the importance of establishing infant-feeding policies and guidelines which are agreed by all concerned.

Help and constructive support may also come from friends or relatives who have breast-fed their own babies and there are a number of support groups which give help and advice to breast-feeding mothers. These include the National Childbirth Trust and the La Leche League.

The family attitude to breast-feeding is very important for its success. An unsupportive father or sceptical grandparent can stop a mother from breast-feeding. If the mother is overtired or stressed, this will reduce the supply of milk.

A common reason for stopping breast-feeding is the belief that the milk has 'dried up'. There does seem to be a relative dip in milk production after a few weeks in some cases, resulting in an increased demand by the baby to be fed. This can often be overcome by suckling the baby more frequently to increase stimulation, ensuring that the mother is getting enough rest and that she has an adequate fluid intake.

During the last five years, after a rapid rise in breast-feeding nationally, the proportion of mothers who breast-feed their babies has stabilized at around 40 per cent at six weeks, and it is possible that the rate of breast-feeding is beginning to decline again. Most of the mothers who are not breast-feeding at this stage chose from the beginning not to do so. It is also likely that a significant proportion of mothers who begin to breast-feed and then give up were not fully committed from the start and use whatever pretext is at hand to switch to the bottle.

It appears that there is a hard core of mothers not predisposed to breast-feeding their babies. Whether the present plateau in the number of breast-feeding mothers is permanent, a pause before a further increase, or a prelude to decline, time alone will tell. Contrary to some views we think that the problem arises not from what happens after the mother becomes pregnant or after the baby is born, but from attitudes established long before these events. Women who are determined to breast-feed usually succeed. Although it is important that mothers who start breast-feeding their babies should be given all the support and advice they need, it seems that those who favour more breast-feeding (most health professionals) will need to concentrate their efforts on educating the young would-be parents from less-privileged social-class groups into believing that it is desirable.

Establishing lactation

Fixation

Newborn infants are endowed with surprisingly little innate behaviour, and most of this we share with our primate cousins. It consists mainly of survival reflexes such as head turning, startle, and grasp. Among these are reflexes associated with feeding—the ability to suck and swallow, and the rooting reflex. These are present in all but the more preterm newborn infants. Curiously, the ability to fix at the nipple does not appear to be inborn and infants vary considerably in the speed with which they learn the trick. This is to a considerable extent determined by the skill of the person who assists the mother with the first feeds.

Successful fixing appears to be influenced by other factors:

1. The state of mind of the mother.
2. The degree of alertness of the baby.
3. The condition of the nipples.
4. The timing of the first feed.

Above all it depends on understanding how the baby fixes, not by grasping the nipple but by drawing the nipple, together with a part of the areolar breast tissue, into its mouth.

A difficult struggle at this time can have a devastating effect on the mother's morale and may be an important determining factor in later success of lactation. Borderline potential breast-feeders may well swing towards artificial feeding if the initial experience is unpleasant. A gentle and supportive assistant can make all the difference. It has been suggested that voluntary agencies have a role to play in this but there has always been some resistance to this idea among professionals. It is also questionable whether the lying-in wards of busy maternity units are the ideal place for this delicate and personal event. Fortunately most babies are obliging, learn quickly, and are soon adept at the art.

The first days

At birth, milk production is close to zero because of the inhibiting effect of placental oestrogen. The removal of the placenta results in a sudden stimulus to production of colostrum but the volume is very low. The energy content is well below even the lower needs of the newborn infant (see Fig. 1.1). The metabolic rate of newborn infants is low but increases rapidly during the first week of life so that energy consumption almost doubles. It is thus inevitable that breast-fed babies will lose some weight during the first days of life. The colostrum is of course very useful for its antibody content and the presence of other humoral agents. The very low energy intake acts as a feeding stimulus to the baby, who will be predisposed to suck vigorously when put to the breast. This in turn acts as an important stimulus to increasing milk production, first by leading to the release of

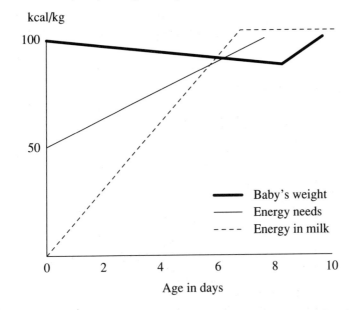

Fig. 1.1. Schematic representation of energy balance during the first days of life.

oxytocin, which causes contraction of myo-epithelial cells in the milk ducts propelling milk out of the breast, and second, by stimulating production of prolactin, which in turn stimulates the formation and maturation of the milk (Fig. 1.2).

In addition to these direct effects, oxytocin may, by inducing pleasure in the mother, reinforce the desire to breast-feed, while prolactin acts as a suppressor of ovulation. With successful establishment of lactation a supply of milk begins to flow which increases with the needs of the baby. These favourable events presuppose that the healthy, hungry baby will be put to the breast at frequent intervals.

Early weight loss

As has been said some weight loss is inevitable in the breast-fed baby. Mothers should be prepared for this and reassured that no harm will result. The baby should be weighed regularly during the first week, and only if the weight falls significantly is inter-

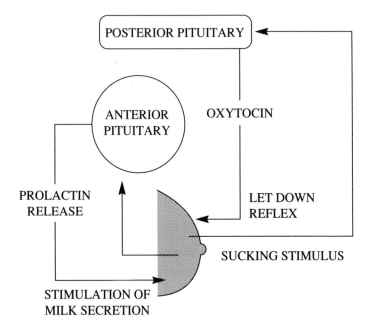

Fig. 1.2. Reflexes involved in the establishment of breast milk secretion.

vention necessary. In the past a weight loss of up to 10 per cent during the first ten days was considered acceptable and, in the fullterm normal-sized infant, there appears to be no reason to depart from this rule of thumb.

Some judgement is required. Occasionally a young baby may become dehydrated because of fever, diarrhoea, vomiting, or hyperventilation. From time to time an infant will lose weight at such a rapid rate that it is obvious that it will lose more than 10 per cent of its weight. The administration of extra fluid or even formula, as a complement rather than a supplement, may be required to prevent malnutrition.

Complements and supplements

There are two alternative ways of providing a breast-fed infant with food other than breast milk. Either the baby can be offered a bottle immediately after a breast-feed (complementary feed) or it can be given a bottle independently of its breast-feeding pattern (supplementary feed).

It cannot be emphasized too strongly that the great majority of breast-fed babies do not require extra feeds and these should only be offered if there is a good reason to do so. There is evidence that giving babies formula during the period in which lactation is being established reduces the likelihood of success. When this is done there is a greatly increased chance that breast-feeding will stop altogether. It interferes with the cycle of hormonal stimulation that ensures maintenance of and increase in milk secretion. The occasional situation where this is justified is discussed in the preceding section.

Although all artificial feeds should be avoided during the early days, if for some reason extra intake is deemed necessary then complementary feeding is far preferable because it does not interfere with the natural rhythm of demand feeding that is hopefully building up between mother and baby.

Colostrum

During the first few days after birth, colostrum is produced by the mammary gland. This protein-rich food has a specific amino-acid composition, very high in arginine and tryptophan. It also has high levels of minerals and particularly vitamins A, D, and B_{12}. The fat content—and therefore its energy content—is much lower than that of mature breast milk.

Much of the protein in colostrum consists of immunoglobulins (mainly IgA), which may have a useful role to play in preventing infection and blocking early introduction of allergens through the gastro-intestinal mucous membranes. Of the three important classes of immunoglobulins, IgG crosses the placenta so that the baby is effectively passively immunized by its mother against those antigens which produce IgG antibodies, whereas IgM does not cross the placenta and is produced by the fetus and the newborn infant. Since IgA is not produced by the very young baby and does not cross the placenta, colostrum, and to an extent mature breast milk, helps to bridge the resulting antibody gap. Colostrum also contains living cells which are capable of releasing antibodies and other agents after ingestion. The presence of an antitrypsin factor prevents the digestion of much of the protein thus allowing the antibodies to survive in the gut during these early days.

Colostrum contains other anti-infective agents, including lysozyme, which inhibits bacterial growth, and lactoferrin, which binds iron in the intestine thus making it unavailable for bacterial growth. It also contains agents which bind other compounds, such as vitamin B_{12} and folate.

The exact importance of these antibodies and antibacterial agents is not clear but it seems prudent to assume that some advantage results from their presence. As the baby matures, it becomes able to produce its own IgA, which is secreted by gut epithelial cells onto the surface of the bowel where it exerts a protective effect. The IgA present in colostrum and also in mature breast milk may be seen as a temporary substitute, filling the time gap during which the baby does not produce its own IgA.

Mature breast milk

Frequent suckling by the infant during the first few days of life not only causes the amount of breast milk to increase but also results in its transformation into mature milk with a gradual change in its nutritional composition. In fact, breast milk is never quite homogeneous, and the initial part of the feed is always more similar to colostrum (the 'fore milk') than the milk secreted as the feed progresses (the 'hind milk'). The composition of so-called mature milk is an averaging out of the transition that occurs within each feed. This 'average' product contains much less protein than colostrum and has a much higher fat and therefore energy content (Table 1.2). It still contains, albeit in lower concentrations, the antibodies and antibacterial agents present in colostrum, although the total amount may not be reduced since the volume is greatly increased.

Human milk contains digestive enzymes, in particular lipase and amylase. These may enable the young infant to absorb the fat and carbohydrate in the milk more effectively. Lipase is considered particularly important since infants depend upon a continuous supply of essential fatty acids and fat to maintain growth and development.

Table 1.2 Composition of mature human milk
(per 100ml)

Component	Human milk
Energy (kcal)	70
Protein (g)	1.3
Lactose (g)	7.0
Fat (g)	4.2
Vitamin (μg)	
A	60
D	0.01
E	0.35
K	0.21
Thiamin	16
Riboflavin	30
Nicotinic acid	230
B_{12}	0.01
B_6	6
Folate, total	5.2
Pantothenic acid	260
Biotin	3.8
C (mg)	3.8
Sodium (mg)	15
Potassium (mg)	60
Chloride (mg)	43
Calcium (mg)	35
Phosphorus (mg)	15
Magnesium (mg)	2.8
Trace elements (μg)	
Iron	76
Copper	39
Zinc	295
Iodine	7

(Adapted from *Present day practice in infant feeding* (DHSS 1987).)

Mature human milk contains approximately 70 kcals/100 ml, of which about 50 per cent is derived from fat (Table 1.2). The remainder is provided by carbohydrate and any protein surplus to growth needs.

Lactose is the carbohydrate in milk. It is a disaccharide consisting of two monosaccharides, glucose and galactose. Before it can be absorbed, it is digested in the small bowel (the jejunum) by the enzyme lactase. This enzyme, as we shall see, is very vulnerable, and defects in lactase are a relatively common cause of nutritional problems.

Human milk contains all the vitamins, minerals, and trace elements known to be essential for the infant's needs, provided that an adequate volume of milk is taken and that the mother's diet is satisfactory. It sometimes appears at first glance that the concentrations of certain substances are low but two factors have to be taken into account: first, the 'bio-availability' (efficiency of absorption) of a mineral such as iron is very high in human milk and second, there are a number of substances, i.e. copper, iron, and certain vitamins, that are built up during later pregnancy and supplement the baby's supply during the first months of life. Premature babies and infants from some ethnic groups (e.g. Asians) do not receive these stores and may be more likely to become deficient.

Drugs in breast milk

Most drugs taken by the mother during lactation either do not harm the baby or pass into breast milk in such low concentrations that they are harmless. Nevertheless care should be taken regarding drugs prescribed to the lactating mother. The British National Formulary carries an excellent and authoritative review of the relative risks of drugs which may pass into breast milk. We describe here those which are listed as 'best avoided' and the possible harmful effects they may have. We also give some commonly prescribed drugs which are known to be safe. However, since the list of drugs and their side-effects is long and growing, it is important always to consult the Formulary before prescribing or taking a drug not mentioned here.

Alcohol is excreted in breast milk and will produce drowsiness in the infant if taken in large amounts.

Of the hormonal drugs, androgens should be avoided because of the virilizing effect they may have on the female infant and the possibility of precocious puberty in the male. The oral contraceptives, which contain oestrogen, may have a suppressant effect on milk formation before the flow has become established. Antithyroid drugs such as carbimazole will reach the infant and may suppress its thyroid gland; propythiouracil is less likely to have this effect. All iodine-containing preparations should be avoided, including topical agents. Corticosteroids in a dose greater than 10 mg per day may cause adrenal suppression in the baby. Oral hypoglycaemic drugs may lower the blood glucose of the infant but insulin does not.

Drugs used for treating constipation, such as the anthroquinones present in senna or cascara, and phenolphthalein, may cause diarrhoea in the baby.

The anticoagulant phenindione causes bleeding in the baby but warfarin is safe.

Possibly the most commonly prescribed drug best avoided is aspirin. It crosses into the breast milk and may on very rare occasions cause Reye's syndrome in a susceptible infant. Paracetemol crosses into breast milk but is not known to be harmful. Of the non-steroidal anti-inflammatory agents, indomethacin is found in high concentrations in breast milk and one case of convulsions has been described. Drugs such as ketobrufen, ibubrufen, and piroxicam are found in amounts too small to be harmful. Care should be exercised in the use of gold, which is found in breast milk and might cause an idiosyncratic drug reaction.

The opiate drugs, particularly heroin (diamorphine) and morphine, are most likely to be present in the breast milk of addict mothers and their presence is therefore not under medical control. It is no longer believed that the best treatment for addicted babies is to receive small quantities of drug in breast milk, and breast-feeding in such cases should be stopped. Mothers on a methadone therapeutic regime can continue to breast-feed.

Ephedrine and pseudo-ephedrine are found in breast milk in significant amounts and the former has been described as a cause of excitation and irritability.

Cytotoxic drugs are an absolute contra-indication to breast-feeding.

Calciferol (vitamin D) and vitamin A in high dosage can be toxic.

Among the most commonly prescribed drugs are the psychotropic agents, sedatives, antidepressants, drugs for mania, and tranquillizers. Since postnatal psychosis and emotional disturbance is not rare, and since many mothers may have been on such drugs before pregnancy, it is important to know which drugs are compatible with continued breast-feeding. The tricyclic antidepressants do not cross into breast milk in sufficient concentration to cause harm. Most antipsychotic drugs are safe, but chlorpromazine may occasionally cause drowsiness and should be used with caution. Meprobamate is specifically concentrated in breast milk and is best avoided. Barbiturates have a sedative effect on the infant and are best avoided. Lithium may continue to be used with caution but maternal blood levels should be monitored since high concentrations may cause intoxication in the baby. The benzodiazepines cause drowsiness and weight loss if used repeatedly. Chloral hydrate will also sedate the infant.

Among commonly used antibacterial drugs, the sulphonamides and preparations containing them, e.g. co-trimoxazole, may cause kernicterus in young infants with jaundice or may precipitate haemolytic anaemia in rare cases where there is a predisposition. Tetracycline carries the theoretical risk of staining the teeth but this may be prevented by chelation with calcium in the breast milk. Chloramphenicol may cause aplastic anaemia and should not be used in a breast-feeding mother. Metranidazole makes the milk bitter and should not be used in high dosage. Nitrofurantoin carries a tiny risk of causing haemolytic anaemia for the same reasons as the sulphonamides.

Certain drugs which cross into breast milk in significant amounts but which cause no harm include most antihistamines (clemastine has been described to cause drowsiness in a baby), cimetadine, ranitidine, erythromycin, ethosuximide, minoxidil, pyrimethamine, quinidine, spironolactone, and trimethoprim.

Other drugs which cross into breast milk in concentrations too low to be harmful include acetozolamide, azathioprine, baclofen, most beta-blockers (infants should be monitored for toxicity), carbamazepine, chlormethiazole, chloroquine, codeine, cycloserine, dextropropoxyphene, diclophenac, digoxin, disopyramide, domperidone, ethambutol, frusemide, halo-

peridol, heparin, hyoscine, loprazolam, methyldopa, nitraze-
pam, phenytoin, rifampicin, terbutaline, and thiazides.

Environmental pollution is another concern. Both artificially
fed and breast-fed babies ingest small quantities of pesticide
residues, although these levels may have fallen recently. There is
no evidence that present levels are harmful, but this is an area
where there is no room for complacency and the addition of
non-biodegradable or slowly degradable residues to the environment should be actively resisted. The Chernobyl disaster has
also raised concern about radioactivity in milk. There is
evidence that breast-fed babies suffered less ingestion of substances such as radioactive iodine than did formula-fed infants.
During periods where there is a risk of radioactive contamination, babies should be breast-fed for as long as possible.

Although water is generally microbiologically safe in Britain,
in certain agricultural areas, run-off of nitrates from fertilizers
may enter the water supply and can pose a danger in some
conditions, such as drought. Lead may be present in water in
higher than acceptable concentrations if the supply pipes are
lead and the water is very soft. Fluoride in water remains an
emotive issue. It poses no threat to either breast- or bottle-fed
infants. Fluoridation of water supplies where the levels are
below average is harmless and should be advocated as a sensible
preventive measure. There is little doubt that it will reduce the
prevalence of dental caries, which although falling for a number
of reasons is still too high.

Mothers who are infected with the human immunodeficiency
virus (HIV-positive), which causes acquired immune deficiency
syndrome (AIDS), should probably not breast-feed their babies,
since there is evidence that the virus can cause infection by this
path. In Britain at present, only a few women are likely to be
infected and many of those are unlikely to wish to breast-feed
their babies. Those particularly at risk are intravenous drug
users, prostitutes, and those with bisexual partners. Most babies
born to HIV-positive mothers are likely to have been infected *in
utero*. In the developing world in countries where large numbers
of women are now HIV-positive, breast-feeding may be far the
lesser of two evils.

Maternal diet during pregnancy and lactation

Good nutrition and a well-balanced diet are important before conception, during pregnancy and during lactation, for the well-being of both the mother and the child. Little is known about the effects of preconceptual nutrition on the development of the fetus but a varied diet is desirable with adequate energy intake and a balance of all nutrients. There is some evidence that vitamin intake at conception and soon after may be important in preventing certain congenital anomalies, particularly spina bifida. Although the findings have not been tested in a double-blind study as yet, there seems no reason why potential mothers should not ensure that there is an adequate intake of vitamins in their diet. Vitamin supplements should only be prescribed if there is doubt about the content of the diet.

Alcohol should be either avoided entirely or reduced to an intake not exceeding the recommended allowance. For a non-pregnant woman this is not more than two glasses of wine or its equivalent per day, and during pregnancy the intake should be less than this. Alcoholism is associated with a pattern of congenital abnormalities so characteristic that it is called the fetal-alcohol syndrome.

Since many women will not realize that they are pregnant for several weeks, preconceptual diet will necessarily be the same for the early part of pregnancy.

During the second and third trimesters of pregnancy, rapid growth of the fetus imposes increased nutritional demands on the mother. The exact requirements vary with each individual and the Recommended Daily Allowances (RDAs) can be used as a general guide. Extra energy is required because of the needs of the growing conceptus and also because during pregnancy there is an increase in fat stores which are subsequently available for lactation. However, as many women reduce their activity and therefore energy expenditure they do not need to increase their energy intake dramatically. It is calculated that an extra 10 per cent increase is required when physical activity remains the same. The best guide is to base energy needs on the rate of weight gain.

Although protein requirement is high, most average British diets provide more than adequate amounts. Protein is particularly important during the last eight to nine weeks since the fetus lays down about two-thirds of its total body nitrogen and tissue protein during this period.

During the last trimester the fetus will also lay down stores of vitamins and minerals, which are important during the early months of post-uterine life (Fig. 1.3). This is illustrated by the deficiency states which can occur in pre-term babies who do not have these reserves. Therefore the diet of the mother should contain enough vitamins and minerals to meet this increased need. Specific examples of this phenomenon are discussed in relevant sections. In certain groups who are specially at risk of dietary deficiency, vitamin supplementation is desirable, for example, vitamin D in Asian women. Women who smoke, an undesirable habit during pregnancy for many reasons, may need extra vitamin C due to the reduced absorption of ascorbic acid.

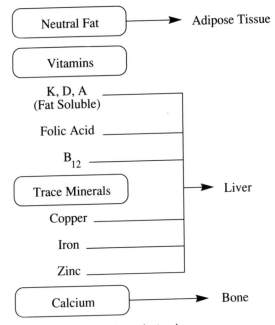

Fig. 1.3. Nutrient storage by fetus during later pregnancy.

Of minerals, iron, calcium, and copper demands are all greatly increased, partly because they are incorporated in fetal tissues and partly in the case of iron and copper because they are stored in the liver. Additionally, the expansion of the number of red blood cells in the mother increases the demand for iron. In women with good iron reserves, this increased demand is met by including high-iron foods such as liver, kidney, red meat, pulses, and green leaf vegetables. This should be accompanied by foods containing nutrients which aid the absorption of iron, such as vitamin C and folic acid.

Extra calcium intake can be achieved provided the diet contains sufficient vitamin D or there is adequate exposure to sunlight. High-fibre diets in themselves desirable during pregnancy may reduce absorption of calcium. It is thus essential that at least 800 mg of calcium is consumed daily (for food equivalents see Table 1.3).

Table 1.3. Some examples of food rich in calcium

Food	Portion size providing 500 mg calcium
Milk	400 ml (2/3 pint)
Cheese	60 g (2 oz)
Yoghurt	280 g (2–2½ small cartons)
Sardines (tinned)	90 gram (3 oz)

The maternal diet during lactation should provide increased quantities of a normal and varied diet based on healthy eating principles to meet increased requirements. For example, calcium requirements are increased from about 600 to 1200 mg. This can be met by including foods rich in calcium such as milk, cheese, yoghurt and tinned fish in the diet (Table 1.3). The alternative is to provide calcium as a supplement. There is also an increased requirement for vitamins A, D, and C, and supplements may be advisable. If the extra energy required is met from foods which contain a proper balance of nutrients, supplementation should not be necessary.

Fluid intake during lactation will in effect be maintained by the normal thirst mechanisms and there is no particular need to deliberately increase fluid intake.

Sometimes substances, other than drugs, present in food may have an untoward effect on the baby. It is claimed that very spicy foods or orange juice can produce loose stools. While such effects are not harmful it may be sensible to avoid offending foods if they cause concern, provided this does not have an effect on overall dietary needs. Occasionally, allergens may reach the baby in the breast milk and if there is good evidence that the baby is reacting to them, then the offending food should be avoided. Care should be taken to ensure that the problem is genuinely due to the food and not to some other cause.

Supplementary vitamins

Whether breast-fed babies should receive supplementary vitamins is controversial. The official recommendation is that vitamins A, D, and C should be given to breast-fed infants from one month of age unless the mother's diet is known to be nutritionally adequate. The difficulty in this recommendation is establishing that the diet is nutritionally adequate, something that can only be ensured by a detailed dietary history. No other vitamin supplements are required unless the mother or baby are known to have some specific deficiency.

The standard vitamin supplement available through health clinics contains adequate levels of vitamins A, D, and C (Table 1.4). If the mother is insistent that she does not wish to give the baby a vitamin supplement and it is suspected that her diet may not be adequate, then a full dietary assessment by a qualified dietitian is necessary.

How long should mothers breast-feed?

Mothers should be encouraged to breast-feed their babies as long as possible and at least until the baby is weaned, but there is no reason why it should not continue thereafter. Breast milk will provide adequate nutrition for all fully breast-fed babies until 5–6 months of age. Thereafter in a significant proportion of infants weight gain will slacken, hence the need for the introduction of solids at this stage.

Table 1.4. Welfare vitamins

Five drops contain:	
Vitamin A	200 μg
Vitamin D	7 μg
Vitamin C	20 μg

Bottle-feeding

In developed countries, bottle-feeding is generally a safe and satisfactory alternative to breast-feeding provided that an approved infant formula is used. These formulas attempt to mimic as far as possible the composition of mature human milk but they cannot mirror its complex immunological and enzyme content. Nor do they necessarily have similar amino acid or fatty acid composition.

Despite these qualifications, if a mother chooses to bottle-feed her baby she can rest assured that there are available perfectly adequate feeds from a nutritional point of view. The guidelines for what constitutes an infant formula are laid down by the Government in line with European Community regulations.

Most infant formulas are based on cows' milk and fall into two main categories, whey-based and casein-based. Casein-based formulas are essentially diluted cows' milk to which nutrients are added but the ratio of casein to whey protein is similar to that of cows' milk. Whey-based formulas are more highly modified and have whey protein added so that the casein-to-whey ratio is more like that of human milk. Since whey protein contains more essential amino acids than casein it is possible to achieve lower protein levels in whey-based formulas. Each baby-food manufacturer tends to produce one whey-based and one casein-based formula (Table 1.5).

The carbohydrate present in most infant formulas is lactose, as in cows' milk and human milk, but other carbohydrates such as maltodextrin are permitted. All these formulas have a similar nutritional content and are all satisfactory infant feeds. Any other milk-based product which does not meet the criterion of a baby food is considered unsuitable as an infant formula. These include unmodified cows' milk, evaporated milk, goats' milk, ewes' milk and unmodified soya 'milk'.

Bottle-fed infants should be demand fed in much the same way as breast-fed infants, enabling them to regulate their own volume of intake. An average intake of 150–200 ml/kg/day is a useful guideline but it is important to remember that babies differ greatly in their requirements. From about the age of 6 weeks, babies develop an internal sensor which enables them to control their caloric intake, provided the feed is made up to the correct caloric density, i.e. neither too concentrated nor too dilute.

The total volume of feed may be divided in six, seven or eight feeds as appropriate. The exact timing and number of feeds is usually dictated by the individual infant, young babies usually demanding seven to eight feeds per day. The number of feeds per day falls gradually as the infant becomes larger. The first feed to be dropped is usually the night feed. The baby then gradually goes longer before demanding to be fed; at about 2 months many infants are feeding approximately every four hours without a night feed. They thus obtain their full requirements from about five to six feeds per day. If a baby is offered too few feeds for its age or maturity, it may not be able to cope with the increased feed volume needed to maintain nutrition. The average number of feeds and volumes of feeds at different ages is summarized in Table 1.6. It should be emphasized that these are averages and that babies show considerable individual variations in their needs.

The formulas should be mixed exactly according to the manufacturers' instructions. In the UK this is standardized to one level scoop of formula powder to 30 ml (1 fluid ounce) of water. The water should be boiled and allowed to cool slightly before mixing. Only the standard scoop provided should be used. Dramatic alterations in the concentration of the formula may result from compression of the powder in the scoop or by using heaped scoops. Over-concentration of the feed may lead to hypernatraemia (raised serum sodium) with dehydration and this can lead to severe brain damage or death. Much of this danger has been reduced since the introduction of highly modi-

Table 1.5. Composition of infant formulas, cows' milk, and follow-on formula

Per 100 ml	Whey-based formulas				Casein-based formulas					
	Premium (Cow & Gate)	Farley's Ostermilk	Milupa Aptamil	Wyeth Gold Cap SMA	Plus (Cow & Gate)	Farley's Ostermilk Two	Milupa Milumil	Wyeth White Cap	Cows' milk	Wyeth Progress
Energy (kcal)	66	68	67	65	66	65	69	65	65	65
Protein (g)	1.5	1.45	1.5	1.5	1.9	1.7	1.9	1.5	3.4	2.9
Casein (%)	40	40	40	40	80	77	80	82	82	40
Whey (%)	60	60	60	60	20	33	20	18	18	60
Fat (g)	3.6	3.8	3.6	3.6	3.4	2.6	3.1	3.6	3.8	2.6
Saturated fat (%)	41.1	39.5	51.8	46.7	41.1	39.5	53.5	46.7	63.2	44.6
Unsaturated fat (%)	56.2	60.5	48.2	53.1	56.2	60.5	46.5	53.1	36.6	55.4
Carbohydrate (g)	7.3	7.3	7.3	7.2	7.3	9.1	8.4	7.2	4.8	8.0
	Lactose	Lactose	Lactose	Lactose	Lactose	Lactose + maltodextrin	Lactose maltodextrin amylose	Lactose	Lactose	Lactose maltodextrin
Sodium (mg)	18	19	18	15	25	25	24	20	50	35
Potassium (mg)	65	·57	85	56	100	70	85	74	150	105

Chloride (mg)	40	45	38	40	60	56	44	47	95	75
Calcium (mg)	54	35	59	44	85	61	71	56	120	115
Magnesium (mg)	5.0	5.2	6.5	5.3	7.0	6.0	4.1	7.0	12	9.4
Phosphorus (mg)	27	29	35	33	55	49	55	44	95	94
Iron (mg)	0.5	0.65	0.7	0.67	0.5	0.65	0.7	0.67	0.05	1.2
Copper (μg)	40	43	46	50	40	39	19	50	20	60
Manganese (μg)	7	3.4	4.2	16	7	3.3	16	11	3.0	20
Zinc (μg)	400	350	400	370	400	330	224	370	360	430
Iodine (μg)	7.0	4.5	4.0	6.9	7.0	10	2.1	3.4	30	7.0
Vitamin A (μg)	80	100	60.5	79	80	97	61	79	40	90
Vitamin D (μg)	1.1	1.0	1.0	1.05	1.1	1.0	1.0	1.05	0.02	1.2
Vitamin E (μg)	1.1	0.48	0.7	0.64	1.1	0.46	0.6	0.64	0.09	1.08
Vitamin K (μg)	5.0	2.7	4.0	5.8	5.0	2.6	4.0	5.8	6.0	6.6
Vitamin B_1 (μg)	40	42	40.3	80	40	39	40	80	40	81
Vitamin B_2 (μg)	100	55	50.7	110	100	53	50	110	200	120
Niacin (μg)	400	690	400	1000	400	650	400	1000	80	610
Vitamin B_6 (μg)	40	35	30.3	51	40	33	30	50	40	48
Vitamin B_{12} (μg)	0.2	0.14	0.16	0.11	0.2	0.13	0.15	0.11	0.3	0.12
Folic acid (μg)	10.0	3.4	10.1	5.3	10.0	3.2	10.0	5.3	5.0	6.0
Pantothenic acid (μg)	300	230	400	210	300	220	400	210	360	240
Biotin (μg)	1.5	1.0	1.1	1.5	1.5	0.97	1.1	1.5	2.1	1.71
Vitamin C (μg)	8.0	6.9	6.0	5.8	8.0	6.4	6.0	5.8	1.5	6.6

Table 1.6. Average number and volume of feeds at different ages

Approximate age of feeds	Approximate feed volume (single feed) (ml)	Number
1–2 weeks	50–70	7–8
2–6 weeks	75–110	6–7
2 months	110–180	5–6
3 months	170–220	5
6 months	220–240	4

These figures are merely for guidance. Many babies will vary the volume ingested from day to day and from feed to feed.

fied infant formula but it has not been entirely eliminated. It is possible that inappropriate caloric density may 'confuse' the internal sensor mechanism and cause overfeeding and subsequent obesity (see chapters 4 and 8). Over-dilute feeds may lead to excessive volumes being ingested in order that the caloric requirement is met. This may cause vomiting. Failure to thrive and malnutrition may ensue because the capacity of the young infant's stomach cannot cope with the much larger volumes of feed required to maintain nutrition.

The need for vitamin supplementation of bottle-fed babies is discussed in Chapter 6.

Partly because bottle-fed babies do not have the degree of immunological protection of breast-fed babies and partly because of the potential risk of contamination, hygiene during the preparation of feeds is of the utmost importance. All feeding equipment and any utensils used during the mixing of the feed must be sterilized. The simplest and most widely used method of sterilization is the use of proprietary sterilizing agents such as Milton, Boots, or Maws. These usually contain hypochlorite solution, and equipment should be immersed for the specified period.

Feeds can be mixed for a full 24-hour period, provided they are stored in a refrigerator. The feed should be removed immediately prior to feeding and warmed to at least room temperature before feeding the baby. Prolonged standing of the feed in a warm environment such as a bottle warmer, near a fire, or on a radiator will create the ideal medium for bacterial growth and should be actively discouraged. Once the feed has been warmed for use it should not be returned to the refrigerator for reuse. Using a microwave oven to warm feeds in the bottle is a dangerous practice because milk in the centre of the bottle may be very hot, and if not noticed it may scald the baby.

Drinks

Extra drinks of fruit juice or boiled water should not generally be encouraged for either breast-fed or bottle-fed babies, particularly during the first two weeks of life because they will interfere with the establishment of feeding. It is not usually necessary to give breast-fed infants any drinks at all.

If a bottle-fed infant is thirsty or cries between feeds particularly in hot weather, drinks of cool, boiled water should be offered. Fruit juices should not be offered before six weeks and are not necessary thereafter. All fruit juices and baby drinks contain glucose or fructose. These, although less harmful than sucrose, do cause dental caries. They should be used very infrequently and well diluted. Dummies and comforters should never be dipped in concentrated fruit juice.

Introduction of cows' milk

Breast milk or infant formula should be the sole liquid feed until at least 6 months of age. There is a good case for continuing these until the child is 1 year old. A follow-up milk may be used after six months. Cows' milk is not recommended until the baby is 1 year old as it has a high solute load, and is too low in some vitamins and minerals—notably iron—which becomes important from about six months when antenatal stores have been consumed. Also, cows' milk is more likely to be contaminated by bacteria than feeds prepared from formulas.

The main difference between follow-up milks and infant formulas is their higher protein and sodium content, which makes them unsuitable for infants under 6 months of age (Table 1.5). In our opinion follow-up milks have no real advantage over continued breast-feeding or formula during the second six months and seem to introduce an unnecessary complication.

The main argument in their favour is the fact that they are iron-fortified, giving them an advantage over cows' milk which is not recommended anyway. Skimmed milk and semi-skimmed milks are not suitable for babies under the age of two years (see Chapter 2).

FEEDING WEANLINGS

Weaning is the process which begins when breast- or bottle-feeding starts to be replaced by a mixed diet. The term weaning means to cease to be suckled. Weaning onto solid food should be a gradual process over several weeks and months starting somewhere between 3 and 6 months of age. The exact time will be dictated by the individual infant and mother.

Weaning is necessary when breast milk or infant formula are no longer able to provide adequate nutrition for the growing infant. It also plays an important role in the development of chewing, and there appears to be a fairly critical time for the introduction of solids by six months to ensure normal chewing development and possibly later speech development.

Weaning should start with the introduction of a small quantity of a smooth, bland, gluten-free cereal or pureed fruit without added sugar. The initial offering should be no more than one to two teaspoons which is then gradually increased. This should be offered at one feed initially, usually before the breast- or bottle-feed. Solids should be offered on a strong plastic weaning spoon and should never be added to the bottle. Adding solids to the bottle defeats the purpose of initiating chewing and can lead to excessive caloric density of the feed. Only a small quantity of food should be placed on the spoon. Initially the baby may only take one or two spoonfuls.

Many babies will refuse the first offer of solids and it is important to emphasize the need to persevere but that the baby should under no circumstances be force-fed. If the baby is upset by the first attempt it should immediately be breast- or bottle-fed and another attempt made later. Sometimes solids may be offered during the course of a breast- or bottle-feed, when the baby, having overcome its initial hunger, may show more curiosity about the new food. Mothers should be aware of the need for basic hygiene, for example, the need to wash hands before preparing the food and feeding it to the baby, and the need to keep utensils clean and should also be aware that all equipment used for preparing weaning foods can be sterilized in a similar way to feeding-bottles.

Following the first introduction to solids, a gradual increase in the quantity, the number of solid feeds, and the variety of foods offered should take place. The exact pace will to some extent be dictated by the baby and the confidence of the mother. There are a wide range of proprietary weaning foods available either as ready to feed, or in a dried form requiring the addition of water or milk. Both savoury and sweet flavours should be given, and variety is important in developing the baby's sense of taste and smell. Salt and sugar should never be added to food. Home-made weaning foods can easily be prepared using fresh foods from normal family meals, provided that no salt or sugar have been added. They are brought to the correct consistency using a baby mouli, sieve, food-processor, or liquidizer. Their advantage is that they are cheaper than proprietary foods but they are less convenient. The amount of milk taken will gradually fall as the solid food intake rises. The changes in feeding which occur during weaning are illustrated by the sample menus in Table 1.7.

By the age of 6 months, babies may be ready to start some finger feeding. They should be offered a small finger of toast, a rusk or a small piece of hard fruit and allowed to experiment with it. The baby should not be left alone with these but should be encouraged to feed itself, however messy the outcome. A gradual introduction of more solid foods and lumpy foods will take place until by one year the child will be taking a variety of solid foods. The infant should be introduced to a cup for liquids.

Emphasis should be placed on the desirability of avoiding sweet biscuits, chocolates, and sweets because of the risk of dental caries. Frequent drinks of fruit juice, squashes and fizzy drinks are also deleterious to the teeth. Fresh fruit, crackers, or bread should be offered if the baby is hungry between meals.

At one year of age, cows' milk can be introduced as a drink.

Table 1.7. Weaning menus[1]

	4–5 months	5–6 months
On waking	Breast- or bottle-feed	Breast- or bottle-feed
Morning	Baby rice mixed with formula Breast- or bottle-feed	Baby cereal mixed with formula Breast- or bottle-feed
Early afternoon	Breast- or bottle-feed	Lunch—fruit or vegetable puree, or ½–1 tin/jar of baby food, or 4–6 teaspoons dried baby food[2] Drink of cooled boiled water or diluted fruit-juice
Tea-time	Fruit or vegetable puree, or commercial baby food Breast- or bottle-feed	Mashed potato and gravy, or mashed banana, or ½–1 tin/jar of baby food, or 4–6 teaspoons dried baby food[3] Breast- or bottle-feed
Bed-time	Breast- or bottle-feed	Breast- or bottle-feed

	6–9 months	9–12 months
On waking	Breast- or bottle-feed	Drink of diluted fruit-juice, breast- or bottle-feed
Breakfast	Cereal or rusk with milk Breast- or bottle-feed	Breakfast cereal, or egg with wholemeal toast fingers Drink of formula
Lunch	Scrambled egg, or cauliflower cheese, or soup with bread, or savoury junior baby-food Stewed fruit, or yoghurt, or milk pudding, or dessert junior baby-food Drink of cooled boiled water, or diluted fruit-juice	Wholemeal sandwiches, or macaroni cheese, or baked beans on toast, or egg and wholemeal toast Sliced fresh fruit, or yoghurt, or milk pudding Drink of water or diluted fruit-juice
Tea-time	Pureed or minced meat, chicken, or fish, with mashed vegetable or potato Breast- or bottle-feed	Chopped meat or chicken, or flaked fish/fish fingers, with vegetable, rice, or spaghetti Drink of formula or diluted juice
Bed-time	Breast- or bottle-feed	Drink of formula or breast-feed

[1] Taken from "After milk—what's next," a leaflet produced by the British Dietetic Association (Paediatric Group).
[2] Mixed as on packet.

Whole milk should always be recommended and at least one pint per day is necessary to ensure adequate nutrition in an average child in an average family. This issue will be further discussed in Chapter 2.

Weaning the breast-fed baby

There are no differences in principal between breast-fed and bottle-fed weanlings. From about five months it becomes increasingly unlikely that breast milk alone will meet the needs of the infant and it is not possible to know which babies will require solids relatively early. It is important that all babies should be used to some solid intake before that time whether or not they continue to be breast-fed. If mother continues to breast-feed, it is quite possible to wean the baby completely without resort to an infant formula.

FEEDING THE PRETERM INFANT

Although most preterm infants, those who are greater than 1500 g at birth, respond well to breast-feeding or standard infant formulas, very small babies pose certain problems. The placenta is able to transfer nutrients from maternal to fetal blood at a rate much greater than that available in formula or breast milk. It is very difficult to achieve intakes of nutrients by oral feeding which enable the baby to grow at a rate which mimics the intra-uterine situation, because the osmolality of the resultant feed would cause major gastro-intestinal disturbance.

Many preterm babies are breast-fed and some workers have favoured expressed breast milk from banks as a method of feeding when the mother is unable to provide milk. Expressed breast milk from milk banks has also been used both raw and pasteurized. There is much debate as to the suitability of this milk for the preterm infant since its composition varies greatly, pasteurization destroys antibodies, thus undermining one of the main reasons for its use, and because of the dangers of contamination. The advent of AIDS has cast a shadow over these methods.

The alternative is to use formulas, and there are several special preterm formulas available. These provide higher concentrations of some nutrients, particularly energy and protein. Their advantage is that they provide a feed of known composition which is bacteriologically relatively safe. There is currently much research into the nutritional requirements of preterm infants and as yet there is no ideal feed.

2

Healthy eating to prevent adult disease

INTRODUCTION

FAULTY nutrition during early life has been incriminated as a cause of disease during adulthood either because the child has been programmed to unsatisfactory eating habits or as a direct result of the effects of unhealthy food intake during childhood. The main concern in developed countries is that children may consequently be placed at risk of degenerative vascular disease (atherosclerosis) either because the process of atherosclerosis has been started during childhood or because the child has begun to develop one of the risk factors for atherosclerosis. These include hypertension and obesity, which may lead to an increased prevalence of vascular disease during later life.

The topic is one of considerable controversy, and unresolved questions abound. Experts range in opinion from those who still doubt whether diet is a significant factor in the prevalence of vascular disease to those who consider that fundamental changes in the way we feed very young children and even infants is imperative. Some epidemiologists have traced the current high prevalence of vascular disease in Britain, not to excess intake, but to the undernutrition present among children of the working classes during the 1920s and 1930s.

Informed parents may well regard this issue as the most important nutritional question they face in raising their children. They themselves may be attempting to adapt their eating habits to a healthier pattern and will be eager to ensure that their children also benefit. Children are not, however, small adults, and proposals which may be very sensible for adults may have harmful effects on the young child. Most health workers will be familiar with the 'muesli-belt phenomenon' of toddlers who are gaining weight poorly and who have loose stools because they have been placed on diets low in fats and high in fibre. Seemingly sensible actions may have untoward consequences. One needs to keep a perspective. Diet is not the only, or necessarily the most important, factor in the causation of cardiovascular disease. Nor may events in early childhood be a very large factor when compared with the unhealthy lifestyle which can be acquired during later childhood and adolescence. The influence that parents have on their children in other ways may be more important than persuading them to drink skimmed milk. Smoking in the presence of one's children, or allowing one's friends to do so, while simultaneously trying to persuade them to consume huge volumes of high-fibre foods, would not be a sensible way to prevent them getting a coronary in later life.

THE ORIGINS OF ATHEROSCLEROSIS

Atherosclerosis is a degenerative disease of the walls of arteries, particularly the aorta, the coronary arteries, and the cerebral vessels. Cholesterol-rich fatty deposits are characteristic, forming a material called plaque. The complete obstruction of coronary or cerebral vessels, which is the end stage of the process, is often due to thrombosis which deposits on the plaque. Consequently there are two distinct phases to the disease; a long process of plaque formation, which may take place over many years, followed by the acute occlusion due to thrombosis. There is little doubt that in certain individuals who are particularly at risk, atherosclerosis may begin at a very young age. Individuals who are homozygous for familial hypercholesterolaemia may die of coronary occlusion during adolescence. Heavily smoking teenagers have been shown to develop severe atheroslcerosis by early adulthood. Autopsies carried out on very young men killed during the Korean War showed quite advanced atheroma. The question is whether diet is a primary factor in this early disease and how soon will bad diet produce potentially dangerous lesions.

Atherosclerosis has its origins in deposits of fat known as fatty streaks. These streaks have been found in the aortas of young children but not in their coronary arteries. They occur equally commonly in children from populations who do not have a significant incidence of adult atherosclerosis, and appear to be the site of future disease rather than evidence that it is already present. Fatty streaks are apparently reversible. Coronary streaks have been found in pre-adolescents from populations with a high incidence of atherosclerosis, and some authorities regard them as more significant of true early vascular disease and as evidence that risk factors for atheroma are present.

The crucial event in the pathogenesis of atherosclerosis seems to be the conversion of fatty streaks to atheromatous plaque, which begins in later childhood (after 10 years) and during adolescence in 'at risk' groups. There is no convincing evidence that irreversible change occurs before then. There is evidence that eliminating risk factors in individuals with quite advanced atherosclerosis will halt the progression of the disease and reduce the risk of catastrophic events such as stroke or coronary infarction. For example, people who have had a coronary episode, greatly improve their outlook if they change their lifestyles by exercising more, by changing their diets, and by stopping smoking. It is thus not self-evident that dramatic changes in the eating habits of very young children is imperative. It is very important not to lose sight of other preventable factors. Teenage smoking may be a far more serious cause of future vascular disease.

RISK FACTORS FOR ATHEROSCLEROSIS

Deciding the extent to which the diets of children need to be changed requires some knowledge of alleged dietary risk factors for vascular disease and the evidence that they operate from childhood.

The possible interrelationships of risk factors is illustrated in Fig. 2.1. It will be noted that diet plays only a part in the overall picture, but potentially a very important part because its consequences are possibly preventable. This is not the place to

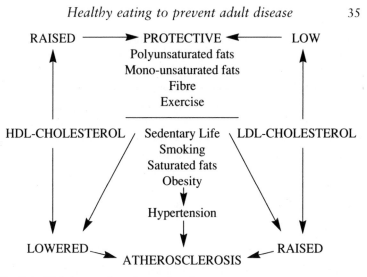

Fig. 2.1. Risk factors for atherosclerosis.

recapitulate the details of the issues involved, but a brief résumé of some of the main points might be useful to the reader. Running through all the considerations is a classical juxta position of 'nature versus nurture' arguments.

Obesity

For many years it has been recognized that adult obesity is related to life expectancy, demonstrated by records kept by Life Insurance companies. This relationship appears to exist mainly, but not exclusively, because of the greater incidence of vascular disease in obese people. It is geometrical rather than arithmetical; the risks rise dramatically with increasing obesity. Someone who is slightly obese has a slightly greater risk of vascular disease whereas someone who is very obese has a much greater risk. The point of 'take-off' seems to be at around 25 per cent excess weight. Not all very fat people have their life expectancy reduced and there may well be sub-groups within the population of fat people who are particularly at risk of atherosclerosis.

The relevance of these facts to child health stems from the fact that many obese children remain fat. It is believed that about 80 per cent of fat children will become fat adults. However, since only about 2 per cent of children are fat, childhood obesity accounts for only a relatively small proportion of fat adults. What is not clear is whether adults who were fat as children are at greater risk of vascular disease than those who became fat in later life. This remains one of the more important unsolved questions. It does seem prudent on balance to assume that it is less desirable to be fat during childhood and that dietary advice for children should discourage excessive weight gain. More is said about these matters in Chapter 8.

Serum lipids

Biologically, man appears to be a hunter-gatherer. Our 'natural diet' was essentially omnivorous, including seeds, berries, and fruits, together with such meat as could be obtained, probably quite rarely. Animals in the wild are generally lean, so such a diet would be relatively high in unsaturated fatty acids and low in saturated fatty acids. Fish-eating people would also be protected by the fatty acid composition of most fish oils. The western diet has tended to move towards a much greater intake of animal fats, partly because we eat more meat and partly because animals reared domestically tend to contain more fat. Such diets have effects on serum lipid levels.

The level of blood cholesterol was one of the first factors to be implicated as a risk factor of atherosclerosis. It is now known that this is not a simple matter, because cholesterol is carried in the plasma in various forms depending on the nature of the neutral fats to which it is attached. The significance of the cholesterol as a risk factor is determined by whether it forms part of low density lipoproteins (LDL)—when the risk is increased —or high density lipoprotein (HDL)—when it is actually reduced. Total cholesterol was originally associated with atherosclerosis because usually high blood cholesterol levels are due to increases in LDL.

Diet is considered important because of evidence that the LDL and HDL fractions can be influenced by dietary intake. Populations on diets which approximate to the 'natural' have low levels of LDL-cholesterol and high levels of HDL-cholesterol. High levels of unsaturated fats in the diet, such as sunflower and certain other vegetable oils, tend to raise HDL-cholesterol and lower LDL-cholesterol levels. Peoples from countries with high intakes of olive oil have low LDL-cholesterol and high HDL-cholesterol levels. This is of particular interest because olive oil is rich in monounsaturated rather than polyunsaturated fatty acids. Some fish oils and therefore fatty fish are also beneficial.

Most other animal fats on the other hand have the reverse effects. Not all vegetable oils are high in unsaturated fatty acids. The so-called 'tropical oils' such as palm oil and coconut oil are little different from animal fats in this respect (see table 2.1). They are very high in saturated fats and their inclusion in many processed foods such as biscuits and cakes or as cooking oils represents a hidden hazard. The label 'vegetable oil' is not a guarantee of satisfactory fatty-acid composition. Even oils which should be rich in polyunsaturated fatty acids may be affected by the process of manufacture. In general, 'cold-pressed' oils are better than those in which some heat extraction method has been used. The repeated heating of vegetable oils rich in polysaturated fatty

Table 2.1. Fatty acid composition of commonly used foods

Food	Saturated (g/100g food)	Monounsaturated (g/100g food)	Polyunsaturated (g/100g food)
Butter	49.0	26.1	2.2
Lard	41.8	41.7	9.0
Margarine (polyunsat)	19.1	15.9	60.2
Suet	56.2	36.6	1.2
Coconut oil	85.2	6.6	1.7
Cottonseed oil	25.6	21.3	48.1
Maize (corn) oil	16.4	29.3	49.3
Olive oil	14.0	69.8	11.2
Palm oil	45.3	41.6	8.3
Peanut oil	18.8	47.9	28.5
Rapeseed oil[1]	5.3–6.6	57–64	25–32
Soya bean oil	14.1	24.3	56.7
Sunflower oil	13.1	31.8	50.0

[1] There are two types of rapeseed oil.

acids will lead to a gradual hydrogenation, turning them into saturated fats.

Diet is not the only factor which influences levels of cholesterol fractions. There appear to be hereditary factors which determine which individuals will increase their LDL-cholesterol levels on unfavorable diets, whereas others can cope with them with impunity. Exercise raises HDL-cholesterol and lowers LDL-cholesterol. Smoking has the opposite effect. Falls in HDL-cholesterol have been demonstrated in teenagers within a few months of commencing smoking. Certain types of personality seem to be associated with adverse blood cholesterol patterns. These additional factors have led at least some experts to doubt whether changing the dietary patterns of the whole population is the best way to tackle the problem of atheroslcerosis, believing that attention should be concentrated on those most at risk.

Some children are particularly at risk. Familial hypercholestero-laemia is a relatively common genetic disorder in which there is no doubt that levels of LDL-cholesterol are raised from early life and that cholesterol lowering regimes are indicated from childhood.

Apart from this specific genetic condition, as with most measur-able indices, there is a range of levels of blood lipids in the general population, which is partly genetically determined. These familial differences can be detected within what is generally regarded as the normal range. This may become apparent from childhood with a tendency for the levels to 'track' into adolescence and adult life. It is on this background of variation that possible exaggerations may occur as a result of environmental factors such as diet, smoking, or sedentary life styles.

Familial hypercholesterolaemia

Type 2A hyperlipidaemia is an autosomal dominant disorder resulting in elevation of the LDL-cholesterol lipid fraction from early life. It is associated with early coronary artery disease. As genetic diseases go it is a common condition. Estimates vary but about 1:500 individuals are likely to be heterozygous for the condition. This means that 1:500 children are at risk of premature vascular disease. This represents a serious public health problem. Because most heterozygotes reach the reproductive age, the chance of a couple both carrying the gene having children is 1:250 000. Thus about one per million of the population will be homozygous with the very severe form of the disease. It is, however, the heterozygous form which constitutes the really significant problem because it is relatively common.

There is good evidence that the onset of disease can be prevented or delayed by lowering the blood cholesterol levels. Curiously, despite the fact that this condition is common and treatable, few screening programmes have been developed, and there appears to be no great pressure to establish them.

At present, identifying children is a random affair, determined by the alertness of individuals. Very few children are actually referred for dietary advice. Yet at the very least, children who have parents, uncles, aunts, or grandparents with vascular disease and hypercholesterolaemia should be quite easy to identify. All relatives of individuals with early-onset atherosclerosis should have serum lipid levels determined.

In the first instance, random blood lipid levels can be carried out. If these are within the normal range for age nothing further needs to be done. If elevated, fasting levels of lipids should be done. Continued elevation of LDL-cholesterol would warrant dietary treatment. The occasional borderline value would indicate a repeat test at six-monthly intervals. The management of hypercholesterolaemia is discussed in Chapter 9.

Salt and hypertension

There is much evidence linking salt intake with the development of hypertension, yet at least in Britain this remains a contentious issue. On balance it appears that certain sub-groups in the population with a genetic predisposition to hypertension are more vulnerable to increased intake of sodium than others, and that limitation of salt intake as recommended by the COMA report is desirable (see below).

Certain ethnic groups, Afro-Caribbean in particular, are at risk of hypertension. This may be because populations who originate from tropical climates have a tendency to retain salt as a protection against losses of sodium in sweat. Hypertension with stroke, rather than atherosclerosis with coronary disease, is the principle risk for black people in the United States. This appears to be related to the high sodium content of the diet. Similarly, in Japan the traditional fish diet, which is high in salt, also appears to increase the prevalence of hypertension, despite a low incidence of atherosclerosis.

On present evidence there does appear to be a good case for recommending that salt intake should be limited for the population at large. Adding salt to food after cooking should be discouraged and individuals particularly at risk should reduce their salt intake.

DIET AND THE GENERAL POPULATION

Policy-making in this field remains a thorny issue. Much depends on the view taken of the early origins of cardiovascular disease. While there is a clear case for placing all children with familial hypercholesterolaemia on a cholesterol-lowering diet with relatively high unsaturated fatty acid intake, greater controversy surrounds the point at which dietary intervention is appropriate to reduce the risk of disease in the general population. The COMA report *Diet and cardiovascular disease* has made recommendations for all individuals over the age of 5 years. These recommendations cover a wide range and represent a prescription for healthy eating (Table 2.2). The recommendations have to be seen in a wider context of suggested modification of life-style, including not smoking (the most important single avoidable risk factor), more exercise, and avoidance of stress.

The reasons for excluding the under-5-year-olds from the recommendations was partly because of the uncertainty regarding

Table 2.2. The Coma Report: Summary of recommendations

---

1. The amount of energy ingested as fat should not exceed 35% of total
2. The ratio of unsaturated to saturated fatty acids should be at least 0.45
3. Obesity should be avoided
4. Fibre in the diet should be increased
5. Salt intake should not rise

These recommendations are not applicable to children under 5 years of age.

the age of the onset of true atherosclerosis, and partly because of the lack of convincing evidence that what happens in the young child is of critical importance. In the absence of compelling arguments, the concerns about the ill-effects of manipulation of lipid intake in the very young was given paramount importance. There remains a body of opinion which argues for the guidelines to be applied to children under 5 years of age.

Some of the COMA recommendations are in fact uncontentious even in the under-5-year-olds. There is general agreement with the view that salt intake should not increase and that obesity should be avoided. The difficulty concerns the levels of fat and fibre which the very young should be allowed and the nature of the fat.

Undoubtedly, a gap exists in the recommendations for healthy eating between the ages of 6 months and 5 years. At the earlier age, most infants will still be receiving the bulk of their food intake either as breast milk or as infant formula. Thus approximately 50 per cent of caloric intake will come from fat. Thereafter there is a progressive reduction in the amount of fat in the diet, with solid foods replacing milk, but there are fears that the type of food eaten by many youngsters will be too high in animal fats. Furthermore if children obtain a substantial amount of their food in a deep-fried form, for example, fried fish and chips, even if the fat used is initially high in polyunsaturated fatty acids these may fall with repeated heating as the fats are hydrogenated.

Although great emphasis has been given to fats high in polyunsaturated fatty acids, such as sunflower oil, there is increasing evidence that diets containing oils with a high content of monounsaturated fatty acids, such as olive oil, are particularly protective. This may account for the apparent benefits of 'Mediterranean-style' diets. The reason for this protective effect appears to be the increase in HDL-cholesterol which such diets engender.

It is probably desirable to continue with breast milk or infant formula until about 1 year of age. This will ensure that a high proportion of the fat intake will be low in saturated fatty acids. The current recommendation is that cows' milk be substituted after one year. If this is done it is not possible immediately to bring the proportion of energy as fat to the 35 per cent recommended for the over 5-year-olds. Nor in the opinion of paediatric dietitians or most paediatricians is it desirable. The problem is that there is a conflict between the recommendation to reduce dietary fat and the fact that many toddlers depend on milk fat for a substantial part of their energy intake. While some households might be able to maintain adequate intake in young children fed skimmed or semi-skimmed milk, there is a real danger that at least some children will become undernourished and deficient in fat-soluble vitamins. Additionally, toddler diarrhoea might well become more frequent: fats delay gastric emptying, and the fall in fat intake which occurs during weaning may cause diarrhoea.

Thus the laudable aim of having similar foods for the whole family founders on the special needs of very young children. Some sort of compromise seems essential if the nutrition of all children is to be safeguarded. The change in fat intake from 50 per cent of energy at 6 months of age to 35 per cent at 5 years of age needs to be accomplished gradually, not by a rapid switch from formula or breast milk to skimmed or semi-skimmed milk, but by a gradual reduction of the proportion of whole milk in the diet. At the same time it is obviously desirable that any non-milk fat should be high in unsaturated fatty acids.

In the United States, the American Heart Association has recommended that the fat intakes of children from 2 years of age should not exceed 30 per cent of total energy. Some paediatricians, as in Britain, have urged caution. There is already evidence that such radical recommendations can cause malnutrition.

After 2 years of age, semi-skimmed milk may be introduced, provided the rest of the diet is properly balanced and the reduction in fat intake is not too drastic. Margarines high in unsaturated fats and uncooked oils such as olive oil on salads should be used and further encouragement of the British public to use these fats is desirable.

Similarly, the recommendation for an increase in the fibre in the diet must take into account the fact that at 6 months of age the diet is essentially fibre-free. It may be very difficult to persuade recalcitrant toddlers to take the very bulky foods that would result if some of the more extreme recommendations are followed.

CAN CHILDREN BE PROGRAMMED TO POOR EATING HABITS?

There have been claims that if babies and young children become habituated to certain eating styles this may be perpetuated as a permanent tendency. Thus children given very sweet foods might develop a lifelong preference for high sucrose foods. Similar ideas have been put forward for salt intake and overall energy consumption. The idea of the 'sweet tooth' conditioned by the nature of food intake prior to the presence of teeth has had wide currency. While young children generally prefer sweet foods, there is no clear evidence to support the idea that giving babies very sweet food will habituate them to prefer such food for the rest of their lives. It will, however, increase the risk of dental caries and for this reason very sweet foods are not to be encouraged. Introduction to a wide range of foods early in life may help to influence long-term eating habits. A very gradual introduction to a healthy COMA-style diet is to be recommended from weaning until its recommendations are achieved at around 5 years of age. The pattern set at 1 year of age should continue with a very gradual further reduction in fat and increase in fibre, bearing in mind that it is always important to ensure that children have an adequate energy intake.

PRINCIPLES FOR GOOD EATING

By 5 years of age the diet should contain no more than 35 per cent of energy as fat, with a sensible balance between polyunsaturated, mono-unsaturated, and saturated fatty acids. Opinions differ as to the exact ratios to be achieved but certainly saturated fatty acids should not exceed a ratio of 0.45. Some would recommend a lower level. This implies restricting the amount of animal fat and vegetable oils high in saturated fatty acids, such as palm and coconut oil. Excessive intake of polyunsaturated fatty acids should also be avoided and a judicious balance of intake of oil such as sunflower and soya, which are very high in polyunsaturated fats, and olive, which is high in monounsaturated fats, should be the aim. As we have already indicated we believe that between the ages of 2 and 5 the transition should take place gradually, not so much in relation to the proportion of the various fatty acids but in the total amount of fat as energy. For example whereas the 2 year-old should continue to receive whole milk, the rest of the fat intake should comprise the oils and fats listed in Table 2.1 as being high in poly- and monounsaturated fats. Convenience and other processed foods should be carefully scrutinized for the exact composition of their fat content.

Before weaning begins, the diet is essentially fibre-free. The weaning process itself introduces fibre. Foods containing fibre which are suitable for children under 1 year of age are included in the weaning schedule in Chapter 1. Thereafter, introduction of a wider variety of solid foods gradually increases naturally-occurring fibre and should include foods containing both soluble and insoluble fibre (Table 2.3). Pure fibre products such as bran should not be part of a normal child's diet.

It is desirable for children to have energy intakes that meet their needs without establishing patterns of excessive intake. Although, as we have seen elsewhere, caloric intake cannot be

Table 2.3. Examples of foods high in fibre

Wholemeal bread
Weetabix
Shredded wheat
Oats
Wholewheat pasta
Vegetables
   Peas
   Beans
Fruits
Nuts

Oats, beans and pulse vegetables are particularly high in soluble fibre which may be useful in reducing blood cholesterol levels.

Table 2.4. Suitable snack foods for 1–5-year-olds

Milk (whole or semi-skimmed)
Fresh fruit
Wholemeal bread or toast with a polyunsaturated margarine
Sandwiches with fillings such as
   peanut butter
   pure fruit spread
   banana
   lean meat
   cottage cheese
   salad vegetables
   tinned fish
Wholegrain cereals and milk
Yogurt
Muesli bars

---

related directly to obesity in an individual child, there is no doubt that in societies where the overall energy intake is excessive, an increased incidence of obesity results.

Snacks form an important part of the diets of young children and ensure that they do not fall short in their energy intake. They are, however, a two-edged sword as they can lead to an uncontrolled intake of energy. Many of the processed snack foods most popular with children are energy-dense and high in saturated fat, sugar, and salt. Thus while it is desirable for children to have some snacks, care is needed in what is offered. Some example of suitable snacks are given in Table 2.4. It is important to remember that some soft drinks contain high concentrations of energy while being low in nutrients.

We have not given precise recommendations for amounts and nature of foods to be offered because of the great variation in the requirements of children, family preferences, ethnic differences, and the idiosyncratic eating patterns of preschool children. The availability of a wide range of foods within the general principles outlined should ensure a satisfactory intake.

The basis for healthy eating for children should incorporate:

(1) a wide variety of foods;
(2) fats which are high in monounsaturated and polyunsaturated fatty acids but low in saturated fatty acids;

(3) the inclusion of high fibre foods;
(4) a minimal use of salt;
(5) energy and protein intake to meet growth requirements;
(6) adequate intake of vitamins and minerals.

3

Dietary variants

THIS chapter is concerned with two very different types of diet; those where, for one reason or another, individuals choose diets which vary from those usually encountered but which are capable of sustaining adequate nutrition, and various forms of 'cult diet' which are unrelated to traditional forms of variation and which are potentially dangerous.

Many ethnic groups have from time immemorial adapted their food intake according to religious practice or to the availability of certain foods. As a result they have developed cuisines which are both aesthetically satisfying and nutritionally adequate. There is evidence that some ethnic groups have developed evolutionary adaptations to cope with what for others might be diets deficient in certain nutrients. Problems arise when people who are not members of a particular culture or ethnic group adopt eating patterns which they may not entirely understand or for which they are not biologically adapted. Children in particular may develop nutritional deficiencies as a consequence. For these reasons anyone wishing to change drastically their eating habits should seek dietary advice.

Difficulties also occur when people used to a particular range of foods and certain climatic conditions find themselves in an environment very different from that of their homelands. For example, children from the Indian subcontinent living in rural conditions in their homelands usually obtain sufficient vitamin D because of the amount of ultraviolet light to which they are exposed, despite low levels of vitamin D in the diet. The same diet may lead to deficiency in those parts of the world with less sunlight. Advice may be required on how to adapt traditional cooking and eating habits to the available produce in order to achieve a good balance of nutrients, and in some cases dietary (e.g. vitamin) supplementation during infancy, childhood, and pregnancy may be required.

VEGETARIAN DIETS

This general term describes all diets in which the amount and character of animal foods ingested is limited. The more meat and animal products are excluded, the greater the potential risk, particularly to children, of diets which are not carefully planned. In principle the problem to be borne in mind is that vegetables have a lower concentration of proteins than meat or dairy products, and the ratio of essential amino acids is also lower for vegetable proteins than animal proteins. Thus greater volumes of protein-containing foods have to be consumed. This can cause difficulties in small children. Vegetables are also inherently less well supplied with certain nutrients, particularly fat-soluble vitamins. On the other hand a predominantly vegetable diet ensures a possibly healthier intake of unsaturated fatty acids and an adequate intake of fibre, which may be excessive for toddlers.

A vegetarian is 'one who lives wholly or principally on vegetable foods; a person who on principle, abstains from any form of animal food or at least such as is obtained by the destruction of life' (Oxford English Dictionary).

In ascending order of animal protein restriction these are:

1. *Partial vegetarians.* This category includes all those groups who exclude some animal products but not all. For example, some exclude red meat but will eat poultry or fish. Partial vegetarians should have little or no problem in providing a balanced diet for their children. Problems may arise if the child eats the low-protein vegetables and potatoes but refuses the food provided as a substitute for meat, or if milk is not included. The nutrients most likely to be deficient in this group are iron and protein.

2. *Lacto-ovo-vegetarians.* Lacto-ovo-vegetarians avoid all meat, meat products, poultry, and fish. They include milk, milk products, and eggs in the diet, which should include a wide

variety of vegetables, cereals, beans, and pulses, plus milk and eggs. There may be a deficiency of energy and vitamin D.

3. *Lacto-vegetarians.* Lacto-vegetarians avoid all meat, meat products, poultry, fish, and eggs. They do, however, eat milk products and drink milk. The diet should contain generous quantities of high-protein vegetables such as beans, nuts, and pulses, in addition to a variety of other vegetables, cereals, milk, and milk products.

4. *Vegans.* Vegans exclude all animal products from their diets. A vegan diet is usually part of a philosophy of life. The vegan diet can be part of a very healthy life-style but the diets, particularly of young children, and pregnant and lactating women, need to be carefully planned to assure adequate nutritional intake and to avoid serious vitamin and trace element deficiencies. Deficiencies of protein, energy, vitamin B_{12}, calcium, zinc, and fat-soluble vitamins have all been described with poorly planned diets, both in breast-fed babies and young children.

Feeding vegetarian children

It is important to be aware of the fact that children require a higher level of nutrition in relation to their body size than adults, and this should be taken into account in planning vegetarian diets for the young.

Most vegetarians breast-feed their infants and continue breast-feeding well after the introduction of solid foods. This helps to ensure an adequate intake of essential nutrients, provided that the mother's diet is satisfactory. In particular, essential amino acids are supplemented, as well as vitamins and calcium. It is important to ensure that the maternal diet contains vitamin B_{12}, especially if she is a vegan. Supplementation of the diet with vitamin B_{12} may be necessary.

If the infant is not breast-fed then an approved infant formula should be used. Cows' milk, goats' milk and some soya preparations are not suitable as infant feeds. Table 3.1 lists the names of some of the breast-milk substitutes which are used by vegetarian mothers and indicates which are suitable and which

Table 3.1. Milk substitutes used by vegetarians and their suitability for infant feeding

Nutritionally complete (suitable for infants)	Nutritionally incomplete (not suitable for infants under 1 year of age)
Human breast milk[1]	Cows' milk
Cow & Gate Premium	Goats' milk
Cow & Gate Plus	Ewes' milk
Ostermilk	Plamil liquid soya milk[1]
Ostermilk Two	Provamel liquid soya milk[1]
Aptamil	Granose liquid soya milk[1]
Milumil	
Isomil[1]	
Prosobee[1]	
Formula S[1]	
OsterSoy[1]	

[1] Denotes suitability for vegans.

are potentially dangerous. It is important to remember that some infant formulas contain animal fats i.e. SMA and Wysoy and are therefore not acceptable to true vegetarians.

Infants of vegan parents can be fed on soya preparations which are approved infant formulas. There are a number of appropriate feeds now available (see Table 3.1). Homemade soya 'milks' or liquid soya 'milk' purchased from health-food shops should not be used as infant feeds because they do not contain adequate energy, vitamins, or minerals. Goats' milk and ewes' milk are also not suitable feeds for babies because they have a high solute load, and are low in folic acid and vitamins A, D, and C. If unpasteurized, there is always the danger of bacterial contamination. Neither goats' nor ewes' milk are covered by the same hygiene legislation that applies to cows' milk, and are therefore a greater potential source of brucellosis and salmonella infection.

The vegetarian infant should be introduced to solids at the same time as non-vegetarian babies i.e. between 4–5 months of age. Suitable first weaning foods include baby rice, smooth pureed vegetables or fruit (no added salt or sugar). Some proprietary weaning foods are suitable as they contain no meat. The baby should continue to be fed the full quantity of breast or formula feeds. Solids should be gradually increased in the usual way, introducing new tastes and textures. Care should be taken to use energy-rich foods, especially as the child consumes less milk. This can be ensured by mixing formula (milk or soya-based) with solid foods, or adding margarine to vegetables. A mixture of cereals and pulses can be introduced gradually. However, care must be taken not to give the young child too much fibre. Beans and lentils should be well cooked and sieved initially. Beans which are partially cooked or raw may contain toxins such as trypsin inhibitors and haemaglutinins which can cause diarrhoea and vomiting. They are destroyed by boiling for at least ten minutes. Slow cookers will not destroy these toxins.

Finely ground nuts and smooth nut-butters may be introduced but whole nuts should not be offered before the age of two years and then only with caution because of the danger of inhalation. Proprietary baby foods have the advantage of being fortified with vitamins and minerals. Vitamin drops should be given from 1 month to 5 years of age. In vegan babies it is essential to provide extra vitamin B_{12}, which would normally be present in soya infant formulas. Older children may be given Tastex or Barmene, which are rich in vitamin B_{12}. Unfortunately these products are high in sodium and are therefore unsuitable for infants. Grape nuts, Plamil and Protoveg are also high in vitamin B_{12}.

The nutritional difficulties which are associated with vegetarian diets and which increase with degree of restriction of animal foods, arise from the fact that the diet is inevitably bulky and this may lead to undernutrition. Vegan children grow less well than the general population. It is therefore important to continue breast-feeding as long as possible or to use an approved infant formula well past the weaning phase. At least one pint of cows' milk or soya formula per day is desirable until 2 years of age since these will ensure a good source of energy, vitamins, and minerals.

As the child gets older the problem of bulk declines, making it possible to join fully with the normal family meals. Growth should be monitored regularly and if poor growth is noted the first step should be to ensure that the child's diet is nutritionally adequate.

ETHNIC VARIANTS

The United Kingdom is home for many peoples who have migrated over the years from all parts of the world. They have naturally brought their traditional forms of eating with them. Food and eating customs form a major part of their cultural heritage and tradition. In their new surroundings these customs may result in nutritional problems in the children. We outline here the major ethnic dietary variants which may be encountered. Most of the groups are Asian and embrace a number of religions, each with its own pattern of food restrictions. The most important are Hinduism, Islam (Moslems), Jainism, and Sihkism.

Hinduism has at its core the idea of non-violence against any living thing and so abstinence from eating meat or fish is usual and the more orthodox (women particularly) may not eat eggs. Hindus rely on pulses and dairy products for their proteins. Possible nutritional deficiencies are similar to those outlined for vegetarians.

Jainism is an offshoot of Hinduism with similar beliefs and ideas. Most Jains, particularly women, are strict vegetarians and may refuse food which has been cooked in a utensil previously used for cooking meat. Many Jains also avoid what are described as 'hot' foods (lentils, carrots, onions, aubergines, chilli, ginger, dates, eggs, tea, honey, and brown sugar).

Asian Moslems follow the dietary laws laid down in the Koran. They are forbidden to eat pork or any product of the pig, or to eat the blood of any animal. Animals must be slaughtered according to the regulations and a short prayer said to render the meat 'halal'. Foods containing non-halal meats are forbidden. Only fish with fins or scales may be eaten. Alcohol is forbidden.

Sikhs have the fewest dietary restrictions: eggs and meat are permitted, though some Sikhs are vegetarian; pork is not permitted.

Fasting plays a role in the religious life of all groups, but young children are not normally expected to fast.

The lacto-vegetarian diet common to many Asians has been found to be rachitogenic in Britain. Many Asian children have been noted to have florid or subclinical rickets. This is probably the combination of several factors, including low maternal vitamin D intake, low levels of vitamin D in breast milk as a consequence, a low intake of dietary vitamin D, and possibly a high intake of phytate-containing foods which inhibit the absorption of calcium and vitamin D. Late weaning onto a diet low in vitamin D may cause deficiency in later childhood. In the homelands this deficiency is compensated by the synthesis of vitamin D in the skin under the action of ultraviolet light of the sun. The relative lack of sunlight in Britain and the high skin pigmentation of Asian children is probably the main limiting factor. Additionally there is a tendency to late weaning and prolonged breast-feeding, which may limit vitamin D intake. It is of interest that rickets has proved far less common among Afro-Caribbean children, who obtain more vitamin D from their diets.

In view of this problem, dietary recommendations for Asian children should include a vitamin supplement containing vitamin D from 1 month of age until 5 years of age.

Weaning should be encouraged between the ages of 4–6 months using adapted family foods to avoid the problem of proprietary baby foods containing non-halal meat products. There is a tendency for Asian Moslem babies to be kept on milk-based food for too long and this may result in iron deficiency. This is aggravated by the use of cows' milk before 1 year of age. This is partly traditional and partly a result of anxieties about the religious acceptability of baby foods available. Certain of the proprietary weaning foods are suitable and parents should be encouraged to seek them out and use them. They are supplemented with iron. Other iron-containing foods which are acceptable should be encouraged, such as egg yolk, halal beef or lamb—pureed if necessary—and green vegetables. It is also important to encourage foods which aid iron absorption, i.e. those which are high in vitamin C and folate.

Progression onto the normal family diet by approximately 1 year of age is desirable. Much support and advice may be necessary, and the language gap may compound the difficulties of getting acceptance of these different feeding practices.

Rastafarians

Rastafarians usually exclude all meat, fish, and preserved foods from their diets. Some are strict vegans whereas others will drink milk. Eggs are often avoided. Salt and alcohol are not taken. Areas of nutritional concern are in pregnant and lactating women and in young children. Late weaning onto highly starchy foods is common practice and there have been reports of iron deficiency, anaemia, and rickets in Rastafarian children. Those who follow a strict vegan diet may become deficient in vitamin B_{12} and folic acid, particularly if intake of green vegetables is low.

The phenomenon of lactose intolerance, which develops in large numbers of children of Asian and Afro-Caribbean origin, is discussed in Chapter 5.

Other ethnic groups

Orthodox Jews exclude pork, rabbit, shellfish, and eels from their diet. Meat must be ritually slaughtered, and milk and its products must not be taken at the same meal as meat following the biblical proscription against 'seething the kid in its mother's milk'.

For the Chinese, food is an art form and they have no dietary restrictions. The only area for concern may be the high salt content of the diet.

In common with these ethnic groups, the diets of Poles, Italians, and Greek and Turkish Cypriots do not generally create nutritional problems or deficiencies in their children. As we have noted, the 'Mediterranean diet' may be near the ideal (see Chapter 2).

It is important to bear in mind that not all members of ethnic groups follow the dietary restrictions equally, and care should be taken to elucidate the precise nature of the diet and not to take it for granted.

CULT DIETS

Cult diets include such practices as the Zen macrobiotic diet and the diets of fruitarians. Other diets followed for cultural reasons may come into this category. The danger of such diets lies in the exclusion of many foods, which may make a balanced intake of nutrition impossible, particularly in children.

Zen macrobiotic diets

Macrobiotics is a regime based on keeping a balance between the Yin and Yang aspects of life thus achieving optimal spiritual, mental, and physical development. Foods are divided into Yin and Yang and the goal is attained by working through ten levels of diet, gradually eliminating all animal products, fruit, and vegetables. The final diet consists entirely of cereal (usually brown rice). Fluids are also restricted.

In its early stages the diet is not severely nutritionally deficient but during the later stages serious inadequacies leading to deficiency states may be produced. During infancy the baby may be protected by breast-feeding but if this is not possible a grain and seed 'milk' is recommended in the macrobiotic regime. A grain and seed milk is totally unsuitable as an infant feed and will lead to malnutrition. Similar problems will arise on weaning the breast-fed baby onto a macrobiotic regime, and there have been a number of reports of harmful effects, including severe failure to thrive and malnutrition.

Fruitarians

Fruitarian diets are based on fruit and fermented, but cooked, cereals and seeds. Only produce harvested by means which do not damage the plant are eaten. These diets will also produce malnutrition and deficiency disorders in children.

Neither the Zen macrobiotic regime nor the fruitarian diets

can be safely adapted for children. To give children such diets, places their lives and development at risk. In cases where parents insist on so doing, child-abuse protection measures should be invoked. A compromise based on discussion and persuasion should usually result in the devising of a nutrition plan which is acceptable to the parents and is consistent with the child's well-being.

Obsession with 'healthy eating'

As we have seen, the current concern to protect children from the hazards of diet-induced atherosclerosis is not without problems. In some cases the concern may become obsessional, leading to diarrhoea, fat-soluble-vitamin deficiencies and significant undernutrition. This results from the drastic restriction of fat intake and excessive provision of high-fibre foods characterized as the 'muesli-belt syndrome'.

4

Feeding problems in infants

IN young babies a wide range of symptoms occur associated with or ascribed to feeding or digestive processes. For the most part they are not due to serious organic disease and are not amenable to 'medical' treatment. Yet they are a cause of concern to parents, often disturb their lives, and occupy a disproportionate amount of the time of health professionals.

Unfortunately they can lead to emotional disturbance in parents and distort the normal, happy parent–child relationship. They are also a happy hunting ground for theorists, unqualified 'experts', and quacks, who exploit parents real anxieties for either financial gain or in order to further their own reputations. As a consequence there is much misdiagnosis of 'organic' cause, and inappropriate investigation and treatment.

DELAY IN ESTABLISHMENT OF BREAST MILK SUPPLY

Occasionally in a well-motivated mother the breast-milk supply may fail to increase at an appropriate rate. The most usual cause of this is failure of the baby to stimulate the nipple adequately by sucking. This in turn is most likely to occur if the baby is not sufficiently hungry when put to the breast. In some instances psychological factors may be at work which inhibit the various endocrine mechanisms already outlined. In such cases significant weight loss will occur and it will be apparent from plotting on centile charts that the baby is going to lose more than 10 per cent of its birthweight before it begins to gain. In these circumstances, judicious use of complementary feeding, combined with emotional support for the mother should tide the baby over until the milk supply is properly established (see Chapter 1). The essential factor to bear in mind is that the baby should still be hungry when put to the breast.

JAUNDICE

About 10 per cent of normal infants have some degree of jaundice during the neonatal period (first few days of life). This is due to the fact that the activity of the enzyme glucuronyl transferase, normally present in the liver and necessary for the excretion of bilirubin, is sub-optimal in some newborn infants. It usually rises to normal within a few days and the jaundice then disappears. This so-called 'physiological' jaundice is almost never significant in healthy full-term infants, but can be a more serious problem in the sick or premature baby where there is a risk of kernicterus.

In some infants this effect is prolonged so that a mild degree of jaundice persists for several weeks. In the overwhelming majority of infants it clears up with no further problems, but since there are other causes of persisting jaundice the baby ought to be checked by a doctor.

Breast-fed infants are slightly more likely to become jaundiced than formula-fed babies. Breast milk appears to contain a factor which inhibts the transferase enzyme, although the exact mechanism remains obscure. All the evidence suggests that this jaundice is harmless. Some writers have recommended stopping breast-feeding for a while until the jaundice abates. There seems to be no real justification for such a course which is bound to cause some failure to maintain breast-feeding. As long as the infant is otherwise well, no action is required. In particular, babies who develop mild physiological jaundice during the first week should not be offered supplementary feeds on that account.

FEARS ABOUT 'HYPOGLYCAEMIA'

Another reason often cited for supplementary feeding while the breast milk is coming in, is concern that the baby might develop hypoglycaemia as a consequence of starvation. This concern arose from the discovery that babies who are underweight at birth are likely to develop hypoglycaemia if fasted. Such infants need to be fed adequately from soon after birth. They have special problems because they have suffered intra-uterine mal-nutrition and so have reduced stores of glycogen in the liver and less fat than normal. This does not apply to full-term, healthy infants whose livers contain glycogen and who can mobilize their fat stores to meet energy requirements. Provided the baby is being fed whenever it is hungry and is not losing weight excessively, breast-feeding should proceed without supplementation.

BREAST PROBLEMS

Failure to establish the milk supply may result from retraction of the nipple, making it difficult for the baby to attach and to gain sufficient purchase to provide proper stimulation. In the first instance this may cause engorgement but eventually lactation failure will supervene. Proper attention to the breasts during the antenatal period, and the use of nipple shields may avert these difficulties.

Many of the problems encountered may result from a basic misconception about how a baby sucks at the breast. It does not grasp the nipple as a bottle-fed infant would do, but takes the large part of the areola into its mouth. This has led to the idea that breast-feeding is traumatic and that initially the baby should be put to the breast for limited periods so that the nipple can gradually 'get used' to the suckling. This is a recipe for engorgement which results from failure to place the baby at the breast sufficiently frequently or in an insufficiently hungry state. A vicious cycle may then commence, with the areola becoming more difficult to grasp. The infant may then become frustrated, the pain of engorgement making it more difficult for the mother to tolerate the sucking, and trauma results from the infant's increasingly vigorous efforts to obtain milk, with cracking and eventual infection. All this is avoidable if care is taken with the initial phase of establishing lactation (Fig. 4.1).

If congestion and pain do occur, it is important to continue

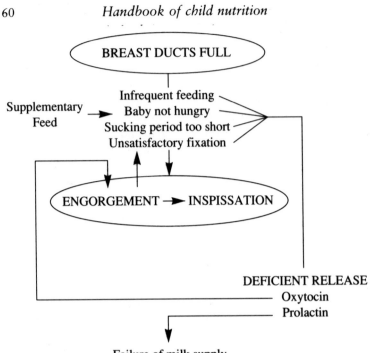

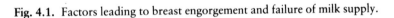

Fig. 4.1. Factors leading to breast engorgement and failure of milk supply.

stimulation of the breast, using analgesics if necessary to minimize pain and discomfort.

POSSITING

Possiting is repeating regurgitation of small quantities of formula or breast milk soon after feeding. It is usually effortless and the amount of food lost is not large. The infants are otherwise well but the effect of persistent dribbling onto clothes and bedclothes may be unpleasant.

Possiting is due to minor incompetence of the sphincter mechanism at the lower end of the oesophagus, allowing liquid food to reflux up into the oesophagus. Characteristically reflux occurs when there is food in the stomach so that the acid gastric juice is diluted, whereas no reflux occurs when the stomach is empty. It is very unlikely that acid juice will enter the oeso-phagus with its attendant risk of oesophagitis. Oesophagitis occurs particularly in hiatus hernia, which is potentially a much more serious but very much rarer condition. Babies who gulp down large quantities of food very quickly may swallow air. This distends the stomach, enlarges the size of the gastric bubble, and reduces the competence of the sphincter.

The sphincter incompetence can be regarded as a form of functional immaturity, and the natural history is for the possit-ing to gradually disappear. In some children it persists well into the first year of life. It often ceases at about 6 months, after the introduction of solids, 8 months, when the child is sitting on its own, or at 1 year, when it has begun to stand.

It is important to have some criteria for deciding whether the symptom is of the usual sort, requiring no special investigation or treatment, or whether it is a significant sign of an hiatus hernia. The following points are helpful.

1. Continued good weight gain.
2. Absence of evidence of oesophageal pain when the stomach is empty.
3. No blood in regurgitated fluid.
4. No pallor.
5. Absence of respiratory symptoms such as paroxysmal cough, wheezing, or choking after feeds, which would suggest inhal-ation, a rare problem associated either with neuromuscular incoordination of the swallowing and breathing mechanisms or vascular ring abnormalities.
6. Failure to respond to conservative management.

Babies who show any of these features should be referred to a paediatrician for further assessment but only a very tiny number of babies who possit require this. It is unlikely that a health visitor will see more than one case of genuine hiatus hernia or swallowing disorder in her career.

It is very tempting to blame possiting on the infant's feed and to use its presence as an excuse for switching from one formula to another. There is no evidence at all to justify this. The only relationship between possiting and food is the fact that by thickening the food the chance of possiting is reduced and this is a recognized method of management.

In cases where the possiting is frequent enough to`be a real nuisance, a careful appraisal of feeding technique may be helpful, ensuring that the baby is not taking too much feed and does not take its feed too quickly thus swallowing air. Sitting the baby up for an hour after feeding will reduce the risk of regurgitation as an effect of gravity.

Feed thickeners

If these measures fail, thickening the bottle-feed with an appropriate thickening agent may alleviate symptoms. Careful consideration should be given to the referral of such cases before further steps are taken.

There are several types of feed thickeners available (see Table 4.1). They can be divided into two main groups:

(1) calorie-free thickeners;

(2) those which provide energy.

In the majority of babies who possit, a calorie-free thickener is most appropriate since the baby is gaining weight well and will not benefit from extra calories. An instant, calorie-free thickener is simple to use and is usually the first choice. Thickeners which require cooking should be prepared carefully following the manufacturers' instructions exactly. In the case of cornflower or arrowroot, the powder should be mixed to a paste with the required volume of boiled water in a clean, preferably sterile pan. The mixture should be brought to the boil, stirring continuously as though making custard. Once the water has thickened, the mixture can be poured into the feeding bottle and topped up to the required volume by adding boiled water. The infant formula powder can then be added and the feed mixed in the usual way. The milk powder is added after cooking to prevent over-concentration and the destruction of heat-labile nutrients.

The feed thickener should be introduced initially at the lower

Table 4.1. Various types of feed thickeners

	Description	Quantity required (per 100ml feed)	Cooking	Comments
Cornflower	Starch 4kcal/gm	1–4g	Yes	Readily available Does not require prescription
Arrowroot	Starch 4kcal/gm	2–4g	Yes	Readily available Does not require prescription
Instant Carobel	Galactomannas gelling agent (from carob bean seeds)	0.5–1g (scoop provided)	No	Mainly non-digestible May cause bulky stools Requires prescription
Nestargel	Hemicellulose gelling agent (from carob bean seeds)	0.5–1g (scoop provided)	No	Mainly non-digestible May cause bulky stools Requires prescription
Bengers	Wheat base Sodium bicarbonate Amylase and trypsin	2–4g	Yes	Readily available High sodium contains gluten Does not require prescription
Gaviscon	Gel of alginic acid Magnesium tricylicate Aluminium hydroxide Sodium bicarbonate	1 sachet	No	High sodium content Requires prescription

concentration and the feed gradually thickened further if necessary. It is important to remember that all the feeding equipment and the utensils used in feed preparation should be sterilized in the usual way. The thickened feed may be too thick for the baby to suck through the usual teat. A larger hole teat should be used or a special teat for thickened feeds.

Bengers (Fisons) may occasionally be useful as a feed thickener. Bengers is a mixture of amylase and trypsin enzymes in wheat base with sodium bicarbonate. It partially digests the feed and will increase the energy content. It has a moderately high sodium content and contains gluten, and should therefore only be used in special situations under strict supervision. The preparation of a Bengers feed is complicated and involves cooking and a timed standing period. It should not be used as a first-choice feed thickener.

Gaviscon is a pharmaceutical preparation which may be helpful in babies who vomit, particularly those with oesophageal reflux or hernia where there is concern that oesophagitis may develop. It is a gel of alginic acid, magnesium tricilicate, aluminium hydroxide, and sodium bicarbonate, and has become one of the most widely used feed thickeners although it is more expensive than others listed. It can be added directly to the feed and does not require cooking. It should not be used as a first choice if a simple feed thickener is required because even the infant Gaviscon raises the sodium content of a feed and could possibly cause hypernatraemia.

Feed thickeners can be used in breast-fed babies usually by offering them as a thick paste on a spoon just before the feed.

In older babies (over 3 months) who possit, early weaning onto solids may be indicated. If possiting persists, a combination of solids and thickened drinks may be useful. The feed thickeners mentioned above can also be used to thicken juices and water. It is, above all, essential to reassure the parents that in the absence of other symptoms this is not a serious condition and will eventually clear up even if they have to wait until the baby's first birthday. Possiting is not a feature of food allergy or intolerance.

VOMITING

The vomiting baby brings back large quantities of gastric contents as a consequence of forceful contraction of the stomach muscles against a closed pylorus. Occasionally the vomiting results from intestinal contents refluxing back into the stomach. Such vomiting will sometimes contain bile and should always trigger immediate referral for assessment because of the possibility of some serious underlying cause. Persistent projectile vomiting, particularly if associated with weight loss or cessation of weight gain may indicate pyloric stenosis. Community health workers should always seek help and advice in such cases.

Almost all babies have the occasional unexplained vomit and the list of possible causes are so extensive that to consider them would almost involve writing a textbook on disorders of the infant.

From a nutritional point of view, vomiting is important for the following reasons:

(1) some vomiting has a nutritional basis;

(2) persistent vomiting may cause undernutrition.

Babies who are overfed may vomit because their gastric capacity is simply too small to cope with the volume of feed taken. Occasionally this increased volume will be an indirect consequence of over-diluted formula, where the baby compensates for the low caloric density of the feed by taking a greater volume.

Food intolerance or allergy may cause vomiting but this is usually associated with diarrhoea and/or poor weight gain or other signs of acute allergy such as skin reactions. If it is suspected that persistent vomiting is due to intolerance, the baby should be referred to a paediatrician. For reasons explained elsewhere, it is a mistake simply to alter the baby's formula without confirmation of the diagnosis.

A persistently vomiting baby is potentially seriously ill and requires careful assessment to exclude other causes of vomiting. It is dangerous to switch formulas in such babies on a speculative basis.

RUMINATION AND HABITUAL VOMITING

Babies may learn to deliberately regurgitate food from the stomach, which they then taste, chew, and re-swallow. Some of the food is inevitably lost in the process through vomiting. The techniques the infants use are either to push the fingers into the mouth and so stimulate the gag reflex, or to use the tongue to produce the same effect. The baby may learn to ruminate only when not being watched. If the food losses are sufficient, failure to thrive may result. Certain babies are likely to develop rumination; they are infants with reflux vomiting, some mentally retarded babies, and those who have been deprived and understimulated when it forms part of the maternal deprivation syndrome.

Management consists of preventing fingers being pushed into the mouth, thickening of feeds, early weaning, distraction of the child after it has been fed, and adequate stimulation.

COLIC

Three-month or evening colic is a common functional condition of young babies, which may be very distressing to the infant and may cause considerable parental anxiety and stress but which is ultimately self-limiting and harmless. Infants, usually between 6 weeks and 3 months of age, have repeated episodes, invariably in the early evening. They cry, often yell, draw up their legs, and show every evidence of spasmodic abdominal pain, suggesting colic, a condition caused by violent contraction of the muscles surrounding any hollow organ such as the intestine. It varies a great deal in severity and duration.

Its cause is basically unknown but there have been attempts to incriminate feeding practices and foods given to babies, with the inevitable tendency to manipulate the baby's diet to try to eliminate symptoms. Various studies have failed to show convincingly that there is a significant nutritional basis to the condition. The fact is that evening colic occurs in breast- and bottle-fed babies, and infants fed either cows' milk or soya-based formulas. It has been suggested that cows' milk based feeds are more likely to be associated with colic than breast or soya formulas, yet babies changed to soya fail to show significant clinical improvement when account is taken of the natural tendency for symptoms to improve with time. It is claimed that breast-feeding mothers reduce colic in their babies if they limit their intake of cows' milk, but the evidence for this is tenuous. Certainly if mothers choose to reduce their own milk intake they should seek dietary advice to ensure that they have an adequate calcium intake.

It has to be admitted that the medical profession has little to offer at present. Old-fashioned remedies such as gripe water, some of which contain alcohol, are worth trying. More recently some mothers have given their babies a fennel drink which has proved useful. The most important role of health professionals may well be that of reassurance that the baby is not seriously ill and that the problem will eventually resolve. Parents who find the condition intolerable may often have other problems which are placing them under stress, and attention should be given to proper support through health visitors and midwives. Above all, the impression that the baby is abnormal in any way should be carefully avoided.

In the absence of more evidence it is difficult to sustain the belief that nutritional changes have much to offer in the management of this annoying condition. There is no justification for switching from one cows' milk based formula to another or for the substitution of a soya-based feed. Colic should not be used as a reason to stop breast-feeding.

WIND

Babies habitually swallow air while feeding. This is particularly likely to occur if the infant takes its feeds too fast or, conversely, if for any reason feeding is slowed down by faulty technique. The resulting excessively large gastric bubble causes distension of the stomach and distress. It can also result in excessive possiting. Some babies just seem to be more 'windy' than others. It is not serious but can lead to distress for both mother and baby. At present, the main danger is that wind will be blamed on the formula and ascribed to 'allergy'.

As with all digestive problems, in the early weeks the principle of correct management is to establish that there is nothing seriously wrong with the baby, to reassure the mother, and to examine the feeding technique. A firm, clear statement that the wind is most unlikely to be due to the nature of the milk may prevent unnecessary switching of feeds or abandonment of breast-feeding.

The teat should be checked to make sure the hole is neither too large nor too small. The method used for mixing the feed should also be checked to make sure it does not include vigorous shaking immediately prior to feeding since this will include many air bubbles into the feed which may be contributing to the problem. The mother should be watched feeding the baby, frequently if air swallowing is a major problem, and advised on how to prevent air swallowing, how to slow down the rate of feeding, and how to 'wind' the baby. Some of the more common mistakes in feeding which contribute to wind include not tilting the bottle correctly, thus allowing the teat to become empty, and not removing the bottle from the baby's mouth at intervals to prevent the teat collapsing. This again encourages the baby to gulp air. If it is difficult to remove the bottle from the baby's mouth during feeding, the use of a bottle with a disposable bag interior may be helpful since this collapses as the baby feeds.

CONSTIPATION

Constipation is a common complaint during infancy. Breast-fed babies are rarely constipated since breast milk tends to have a mildly aperient effect, partly due to the lactose of breast milk being more slowly absorbed than that of artificial feeds because of a subtle difference in the chemical structure of human as opposed to other sources of lactose. Additionally the acid, fermentative stools of the breast-fed baby are softer and more bulky than those of the formula-fed baby. It is not unusual for breast-fed babies to pass many soft stools daily, which the unwary might mistake for diarrhoea, although curiously some infants seem to store it all up for an occasional massive explosive episode.

Parents often become disproportionately anxious about their

babies' bowel habits and often it is reassurance that is required rather than action since the infants are not truly constipated. Artificially fed babies who have at least one stool every other day without excessive straining are unlikely to have serious problems.

Constipation is more common in formula-fed babies but in the absence of organic disease is rarely severe. Stools may be small, greenish, pellet-like, and occasionally these may be blood-streaked if a fissure develops. Fissures are painful and may perpetuate the constipation.

If constipation is a problem in young babies, the first step should be to ensure that an adequate fluid intake is being given. Extra drinks of boiled water can be helpful, as can fruit juices such as pure or fresh orange juice diluted with water. Temporary relief can be obtained by adding some sugar to the bottle; this will give a higher osmolar feed which will draw fluid into the bowel and create a softer stool. Very dilute prune juice has also been found to be helpful.

If a baby is genuinely constipated, the introduction of solids at 3 months of age can help. Pureed fruits, vegetables, and cereals should be encouraged. Wholegrain cereals can be introduced gradually from 6 months of age and beans and pulses at a later stage. Pure bran is not recommended in very young children and is not necessary if the fibre content of the diet is gradually increased using foods naturally high in fibre. It is important to ensure that the infant has a good fluid intake because fibre absorbs water.

Severe constipation with soiling is a problem of the older child and is discussed in Chapter 6.

CHOKING EPISODES

One of the most frightening things that can happen to a parent is to see their young child choke on food. It can happen with either liquid or solids but is particularly likely at the time when the infant is beginning to take solids and may have to deal with a lump which causes it to gag. The occasional child seems to have special difficulty with or aversion to lumpy food and the assistance of a speech therapist or clinical psychologist skilled in the use of desensitization techniques may be helpful.

Sometimes apnoeic episodes, which are quite common in young babies, may be interpreted as choking. It can be very difficult in retrospect to be quite sure what has happened. In either event attempts at reassurance may be the best policy.

There are some important organic disorders which may be associated with choking. Repeated episodes should be treated seriously and warrant referral for further investigation.

'RUNNING OUT OF MILK'

About 25 per cent of infants who appear to be well established on the breast, being demand fed, at about 6–8 weeks of age require to be fed more frequently. The mother will find that during the day particularly, she may have to feed the baby as often as hourly. Interestingly these babies usually continue to sleep well at night.

Unfortunately this can be interpreted by both mother and health adviser as evidence of 'running out of milk' whereas in fact it represents a short term readjustment. The baby may indeed at this point not be getting enough milk and responds in an entirely appropriate way, by demanding to be fed more often. The appropriate parental response should be to feed the baby more frequently. This will quite rapidly lead to further stimulation of the breast to increase the supply of milk and usually within a few days the baby will settle back to a more usual routine. We have found that if this is carefully explained to the mother, she will be willing to accept a more frequent rate of feeding for a limited period—usually less than a week. Offering the baby supplementary feeds at this point will almost certainly result in a reduction of milk supply, further unhappiness from the baby, and eventual cessation of breast-feeding.

The 4–6 week period is often a low point for the mother of a young baby. The initial excitement will have worn off and the drudgery involved in the daily care of the infant may result in increasing tiredness. Both parents will at this point wish to renew their social and other activities, all of which may contribute to a degree of exhaustion. If this is coupled with an inadequate calorie and nutrient intake, it may reflect in either a reduction of milk supply or a failure to increase it in line with the needs of the baby. Continued emotional support and practical help from the father or other family members to reduce the sheer physical activity, together with sensible dietary advice, may prevent many cases of secondary lactation failure.

OVERFEEDING AND UNDERFEEDING

Most babies appear to have an internal caloric sensor which enables them to control the amount of energy they take in. While it is the size of the baby which will determine the average intake there is much variation in the quantity of food that babies require to achieve a normal growth rate. The reasons for this are still not fully understood but there is evidence that underlying rates of metabolism vary. Thus some babies will require as little as 100 ml of formula per kilo per day, whereas others will require as much as 200 ml. Much so-called overfeeding or underfeeding is the result of too rigid application of norms. If a baby is well and growing at a normal rate, too much should not be made of the actual volume of intake.

Concern may arise if a baby is obviously fat. Whether infants should be dieted is a controversial matter discussed in detail in Chapter 8.

Underfeeding should only be considered if a baby is failing to grow along appropriate milestones. Most infants will quickly signal their dissatisfaction if they are not getting enough food.

One exception to this principle is the problem of the underfed breast-fed baby. Problems may arise if the baby is not fed sufficiently frequently. Very young infants may not cope with the consequently larger volumes per feed. While babies should be demand fed (see Chapter 1), there are limits to the size of the gap between feeds which are acceptable. Parents are often anxious about the exact volume of feed their babies should take. Table 1.6 is an attempt to offer an approximate guide to such questions, but it is very important that a flexible attitude be taken to this matter. Rigid adherence to predetermined figures would lead to inappropriate feeding of most babies.

More important is the length of time an infant should be allowed to go without a feed. While it is highly unlikely that a normal baby would come to significant harm, fasts of longer than eight hours under the age of 3 months are undesirable.

ERRORS IN TECHNIQUE IN BOTTLE-FEEDING

Faulty technique in artificially fed babies is a common cause of problems. These are mainly simple mechanical errors.

Size of teat hole

The size of the teat hole can be important. There are hoary old stories about babies being fed with teats with no hole at all and clearly this would have unfortunate consequences! If the hole is too small, feeding will become a struggle, with frustration of both baby and mother. If it is too big, the baby may take its feed too quickly, distending the stomach, causing 'wind', and possibly aggravating colic symptoms.

Bottle propping

Putting a bottle into the mouth of a reclining baby and letting it 'get on with it' is a practice that has long been held in strong disfavour. The main concern has been the risk of aspiration, and certainly it is not safe for a young baby to be left sucking on a bottle unsupervised. There is also a belief that it may lead to dental caries if continued into childhood. Another important objection to this practice is that it deprives the baby of an important period of stimulation, the interaction with the parent which should take place while the baby is being fed.

BABIES WHO ARE DIFFICULT TO FEED

There is a group of babies who appear to have been appropriately managed but who nevertheless prove difficult to feed. Such infants should always be referred to a paediatrician for assessment. They may be suffering from a whole range of organic disorders, including potentially treatable metabolic defects, or may be showing the early signs of neurological dysfunction such as cerebral palsy, and some mentally retarded infants are difficult to feed. Finally there are some babies otherwise normal who appear to have a functional problem with sucking and swallowing which may require the special skills of the speech therapist or clinical psychologist (Fig. 4.2).

Similar feeding difficulties can occur because of parental inadequacies, but by the time the baby comes to medical attention it may be impossible to resolve how the problem began. A careful psychosocial assessment of the family is therefore essential before the root of the problem is ascribed to the child itself. If there is any suggestion that the child might be at risk, the baby should be admitted to hospital. If the problem is less severe, it

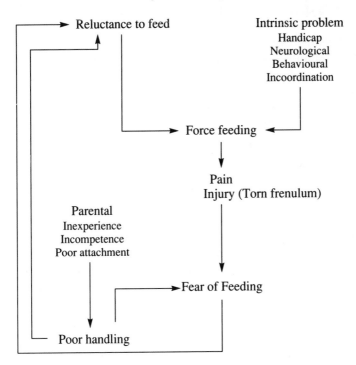

Fig. 4.2. Feeding difficulty in infancy.

may be helpful to have the mother and baby attend a day-care unit where health professionals skilled in infant feeding can attempt to feed the baby and help the mother. This requires skill and tact. The mother's last vestige of confidence may be drained if she sees someone else successfully feeding a baby with whom she has failed.

Whatever the origins, the baby will present as a fractious infant and tends to stiffen and curl up or arch its back when attempts are made at feeding. The baby will either resist the teat being placed in the mouth or simply refuse to suck. If the baby can be induced to feed he may appear to have difficulties with sucking or swallowing, cough, splutter, and choke. The time required to get the infant to take an appropriate volume of feed may be impracticably long, so that virtually the whole day is taken up with the struggle from one bottle to the next. Parents may become exhausted and can be driven to the end of their tether.

The first essential of successful management is to reassure the parents and to show understanding of their difficulties. It may help to explain that this is a common experience and that it will resolve.

It may be appropriate to recommend an alternative teat for the bottle-fed baby who is having difficulty sucking. Sometimes a small soft preterm teat can be helpful, as it may be easier for the baby to feed using this. For the baby who is having difficulties with solids, a change in the type of spoon or in the texture of the solid foods may help. The positioning of the baby during feeding can make it difficult for the baby to swallow or may be aggravating any stiffening or arching. Experimenting with different feeding positions may alleviate this but should be done under professional supervision.

There may also be a behavioural element contributing to the feeding difficulty. In our experience, we have found it helpful to use the expertise of the speech therapist or clinical psychologist to work closely with the paediatrician, dietitian, and parents in preparing a schedule of graduated changes.

Irrespective of the underlying cause, the baby may eventually present a feeding problem to everyone, including experienced professionals, particularly if the parents have reached the force-feeding stage. A short hospital admission may be the quickest way of resolving matters. A period of respite and the calming atmosphere as the baby learns to relax and regains confidence in the feeding process may have a dramatic effect. The mother should be watched feeding the baby so that technical deficiencies can be corrected. She should also watch the baby being fed by others. She may find relief in sharing the difficulty with someone else. On the other hand if the baby feeds well for a nurse, after an initial moment of chagrin, most parents will be enormously relieved to realize that there is nothing fundamentally amiss, and this in itself may enable them to relax with the baby who will respond by being easier to feed.

Observation will also make it possible to diagnose the occasional child who has a genuine functional disorder. Any baby who has a choking episode, becomes blue or obviously tired while feeding, or exhibits genuine distress during a feed warrants further medical investigation.

FORCE-FEEDING

Force-feeding is the end result of several different processes. It is an important and significant symptom, partly because of the direct dangers it holds for the baby and partly because of what it tells us of the mother–child relationship. Its primary cause is the sense in the feeder that the baby is not feeding properly.

This sense may be purely imaginary and may reflect unrealistic expectations of a young, inexperienced mother for her infant. Alternatively, if a good attachment has not formed between mother and baby, tolerance of the infant may be low and any slight 'misdemeanour' by the baby may cause annoyance. The tolerance level may also be reduced if the mother is depressed or unhappy. Sometimes the source of the trouble is not the mother but the fact that many people are feeding the baby, who may come to sense an atmosphere of inconsistency or disorder.

Whatever starts off the process, the effect is similar. The feeder will exert pressure on the bottle, forcing the teat into the baby's mouth. This will induce discomfort and eventually panic.

A vicious cycle may then be set up in which the reluctant or incompetent baby becomes more and more difficult to feed and parental frustration and forceful feeding becomes progressively more intense.

The process of force-feeding will have a number of untoward effects. It will cause the baby to fear feeding because of the discomfort it engenders. The infant may begin to scream at the first sight of the bottle or introduction of the teat. Feeding times will become a real ordeal, and effective feeding may become well nigh impossible, culminating in failure to thrive. A depressed or unhappy mother will feel increasingly incapable and guilty, thus accentuating the emotional upset.

Force-feeding is an important harbinger of non-accidental injury. The frenulum of the tongue or upper lip may be torn and injuries also occur to the palate and fauces. This will lead to extreme pain and screaming and may culminate with more serious non-accidental injury, particularly facial bruising, rib fractures, and shaking injuries. A tell-tale sign is a semicircle of fingertip bruises round the mouth and chin. It is remarkable how common the association is between such external injuries and evidence of force-feeding. If the injuries have been caused by someone other than the mother she may find the whole matter inexplicable, but it has to be recognized that force-feeding may be part of a much more serious pattern of abuse and neglect outside the scope of this volume.

Management is similar to that of any baby who is difficult to feed but there should be no hesitation in admitting the baby, who may be at considerable risk, to hospital.

THE DISSATISFIED BABY

One of the commonest complaints encountered in the early weeks of life is that the baby is dissatisfied with the amount of feed being offered. This is often expressed by the statement that the mother cannot 'fill' the baby. In fact what is being described is really a baby who for some reason either does not settle after a feed or has frequent periods of crying or periods of crying which the mother perceives as excessive. This is less likely to be a problem with breast-fed babies and tends to be a social-class-related phenomenon.

There appears to be a strong correlation with adverse home circumstances and as such is a potentially important warning of more serious problems. Before ascribing these complaints to the baby's feeds, careful assessment of other possible causes should always be made.

Some babies require more food than others. Problems may arise if babies are fed to rigid schedules and parents advised to give fixed quantities of formula. Ideally all babies, breast- or formula-fed, should be fed on demand and given as much food as they will take. Because of the internal calorie sensor mechanism, as long as the feed is correctly prepared, there will be no danger of excessive weight gain. Babies should never be hungry after a feed.

Parents who perceive that their baby is 'not satisfied' may do one of two things. They may either start the baby on solid foods or switch the formula either on their own initiative or on the advice of family or health worker. Some writers argue that there is no harm in this and that realism dictates that these are practices which should simply be accommodated. While the case for some degree of flexibility is desirable it seems very defeatist to accept practices which official recommendations continue to regard as undesirable. There is potential harm to both early introduction of solids and formula switching and in accepting a false explanation for a phenomenon.

EARLY INTRODUCTION OF SOLIDS

During the decade of the 1960s it had become the widely accepted practice to introduce solids at a very early age. Several studies showed that most babies were on solids by 6 weeks of age and in some cases solids were being introduced during the first weeks of life. This was the era of excessive weight gain in early life, hypertonic dehydration, and coeliac disease. This was in part due to the use of formulas based on whole cows' milk and their incorrect preparation, but there is evidence that solids given early formed part of the problem by increasing the caloric density of the feed and by exposing the baby to gluten during a most vulnerable period.

During the first weeks of life, because of the lack of secretor IgA, babies are potentially more vulnerable to sensitization by food allergens and it seems sensible to limit the range of such potential allergens to a minimum.

ADDING SOLIDS TO BOTTLE

In the recent past, thickening the formula with solids had become a widespread practice. Just why some parents do this is not clear but it may be conceived as a simpler way of feeding the baby. The professional objection to the process stems from the increase in caloric density and consequent possible distortion of intake of calories, solute, and water which might result. It also encourages early weaning of the infant which for reasons already stated are considered undesirable.

Another more subtle objection stems from the fact that feeding babies solids with a spoon during early weaning represents an important period of child–parent interaction which may have an important bearing on intellectual and emotional development.

SWITCHING FEEDS

Various studies have shown that in about 20–25 per cent of babies a change of formula occurs during the first 6 weeks of life. This is done for a variety of reasons. In Britain the usual reason given is that the baby was not satisfiedd, whereas in the United States it is usually claimed that the baby was allergic to the cows' milk preparation. Switching of feeds in Britain tends to be from one cows' milk formula to another, whereas in the United States the change is usually from cows' milk formula to soya. This latter tendency is seen increasingly in parts of Britain as well.

Most babies are started on whey-based feeds (see Chapter 1). This is because maternity services generally advocate them as they are most similar to breast milk. There is no theoretical reason why the formula should be changed to any other cows' milk-based feed. Despite this, the rate of switching is high. Since babies are usually on a whey-based feed, the likelihood is that they will be switched to a casein-based feed, something which is reinforced by the widespread belief that babies are less satisfied by whey- than casein-based formulas. Some health professionals actually advocate that babies should be changed to casein-based feeds at 3 months of age. There is no evidence to suggest that this is a sensible belief. Nor is there any evidence to substantiate the view that babies are more easily satisfied by one feed rather another.

Does formula switching matter? It can be argued that as a matter of consumer choice, there is no reason why parents should not shop around among a series of formulas, all approved for use as infant feed, until they find the feed they perceive as satisfactory. This 'free-market' view is open to some criticisms. First there is the philosophical issue that encouragement should not be given to ascribing cause incorrectly. If the baby's symptoms are not due to the nature of the feed it is inherently undesirable to suggest the opposite. The practical aspects of this principle are seen when delay occurs in the diagnosis of genuine disease because the parents abetted by health workers have indulged in a bout of formula swapping (see Table 4.2).

GROWTH PROBLEMS

Whether babies are growing satisfactorily depends on plotting the weight and length on centile charts. Unless this is done

Table 4.2. Examples of conditions mistakenly diagnosed as food intolerance in infancy

Maternal depression
Munchausen-by-proxy
Cystic fibrosis
Hiatus hernia
Child abuse
Cerebral palsy
Renal failure
Congenital heart disease

important errors may result. These charts are compiled from measurements of large numbers of babies. The data is usually cross-sectional when the data at each age are obtained from different sets of infants, rather than longitudinal when the weights at each age are of the same set of babies followed through. The value of centile charts is that infants and children follow a centile line without deviating significantly upwards or downwards along a line presumably genetically predetermined. There are some important qualifications to this assumption.

It is important to use well-constructed centile charts. Some do not include a third centile line. These can be very misleading; babies below the 10th centile, who are quite normal and no cause for concern, may be a source of unnecessary anxiety because they are 'off the bottom line' on the chart.

Centile charts are updated from time to time and it is important to use the latest available data. Some charts have corrections for premature babies. While these charts are valuable for the follow-up of such infants, we have found that they tend to be confusing to those not familiar with them and we advocate the use of the standard charts for routine use.

Centiles for height or length are remarkably consistent and any change in the position of height centile is a matter for remark. This consistency, which has come to be called 'tracking', is probably a reflection of the strong genetic influence on height.

Although weight centiles also tend to track consistently, deviations are more common than for height. This is because short-term effects are more common, environmental influences more powerful, and possibly because the range of weight-gain patterns is intrinsically more variable. This is particularly true for the first 6 months of life.

Normal babies who do not follow centile charts

The newborn infant has spent 9 months in utero, which is a powerfully influential environment. Thus weight at birth is the measurement least likely to reflect genetic predisposition. It is not surprising therefore that some babies show a deviation in weight centiles for a time.

Some infants are relatively small for gestational age. If a baby who was genetically intended to be on the 90th centile has some degree of inter-uterine malnutrition it may be born on the 50th centile for weight. There may then follow a period of very rapid weight gain as the baby 'catches up' to its inherent body mass (see Fig. 4.3). On the other hand, an infant born on the 90th

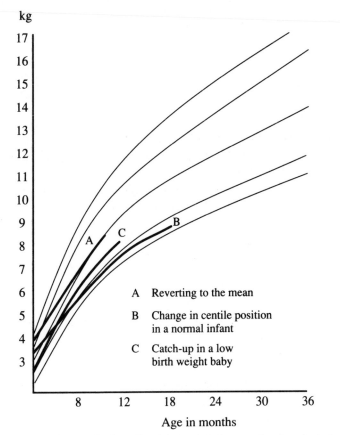

Fig. 4.3. Weight centile chart for girls aged 0–3 years showing deviations from centiles: A, reverting to the mean; B, change in centile position in a normal infant; C, catch-up in a low-birth-weight baby.

centile because some maternal factor has caused it to lay down excess adipose tissue may, in shedding it, lower its centile position.

Because most babies who are small for dates are below the 50th centile and most babies who are large for dates are above it, averaging out these changes for a population tends to show movement upward or downward towards the 50th centile —hence the term 'reverting to the mean', or more properly 'median'. This can be misleading because a baby who is born on the 50th centile who should be on the 90th will 'revert' to the 90th centile whereas an overweight newborn on the 50th centile might, without any detriment, fall to the 3rd.

These factors somewhat complicate the interpretation of centile charts in the early months of life, and it can be difficult to be sure whether one is dealing with a normal reversion phenomenon or a genuine failure to thrive. The great majority of babies who change centiles turn out to be normal. When in doubt it is wise to seek the help of a paediatrician. Usually the best policy in a baby who is in all other respects well is to simply follow and to repeat measurements. If centiles continue to be crossed, further investigation may be indicated, but in the absence of clinical features these are almost invariably negative. One should always bear in mind the possibility that the child may be showing the early features of psycho-social growth failure.

Failure to thrive in breast-fed babies

Breast milk as the exclusive means of feeding infants remains the ideal. Nevertheless there are circumstances in which the amount of milk produced by the mother may be insufficient for the needs of the infants. It is a normal process for the infant's requirements to gradually exceed the ability of the breast to continue to increase supply to meet demand. From about 6 months of age, even in babies fully established on the breast, an increasing proportion of infants will become malnourished if not given some form of dietary supplementation. This was recognized in societies where breast-feeding was universal, in that some solid food would usually be given to the baby from about the fifth month.

The occasional infant fails to thrive because it is not recognized that the baby is not getting enough food from the breast. Characteristically these babies are very quiet and apparently content, and the parents may be unwilling to take them to clinics for regular weighing. Gross failure to thrive can creep up on all concerned. It is remarkable that even experienced professionals fail to notice what is happening and, even when obvious, the diagnosis may actually be rejected by an often tired, depressed, and distraught mother who is deeply committed to breast-feeding and unwilling to accept 'failure'. The emotional reaction can be severe and great care must be taken not to aggravate tension. It is essential, however, to ensure that the baby gets extra feeds, although partial breast-feeding can continue.

As in so many situations in infancy, the solution lies in occasional but regular weighing. It is difficult to see why this should not be done and any reluctance should be gently overcome.

5

Food allergy and intolerance

IN this chapter a distinction is drawn between true food allergy, in which the body immune system has either produced antibodies to particular foods or the tissues react in an abnormal way to particular food or foods, as opposed to food intolerance, in which the harmful effect is not mediated through the immune mechanism but by some basic effect of the food component. The process by which the body develops this reaction is called sensitization, implying that in true food allergy the subject must first come in contact with the offending substance before an adverse reaction can occur.

TRUE FOOD ALLERGY

Immunologically based reactions to food usually occur as part of a tendency to develop allergy to other foreign materials, particularly proteins. This tendency is sometimes described as atopy and is hereditary in most instances. Atopic individuals are at risk of developing eczema, hay fever, acute (type 1) reactions, and asthma. About 10 per cent of the population are potentially allergic, so it is not surprising that allergic conditions, usually mild and often transitory, are common. If both parents are affected then it is highly likely that their children will also develop allergy in one form or another.

One relatively constant finding in atopic people is that they have elevated levels of the protein IgE in their blood. For the purposes of this chapter we will restrict the term 'allergy' to apply only to those conditions in which elevated IgE is a regular feature. All other states will be considered under the term 'food intolerance'.

Not all allergic children have food allergy. Inhaled allergens, such as pollen, animal dander, and the excreta of house dust mites, are actually much more important allergens, causing hay fever, allergic rhinitis, and conjunctivitis, and, most significantly, asthma. Just why children with the same underlying tendency have such varying reactions remains a mystery, but nevertheless a child with one type of allergy is more likely to have or develop another type. For example babies with eczema are quite likely to develop asthma later even if the eczema clears up.

By their nature, food allergens are ingested and absorbed through the intestinal mucosa. There is some evidence that very young babies are most vulnerable to this penetration by unwanted substances because in the first weeks of life a protective protein, IgA, is missing from the bowel secretions and appears in significant amounts only after about 3 months of age. Breast-fed babies obtain some IgA in colostrum and milk, and it may be that this has some protective effect which may delay the onset of allergy until mixed feeding has begun. It may also be that this delay will result in less severe allergy later, because once IgA is present, penetration by allergens is less likely. Exclusive breast-feeding is not however a guarantee that the baby will not develop allergy.

Unless the baby is exclusively breast-fed there may be no benefit, and once the baby starts to have solid foods or other forms of milk, sensitization to those foods will occur. Nevertheless for babies in general and for those from allergic families in particular, it may well be prudent:

(1) to breast-feed exclusively for at least 3 months;
(2) to avoid early introductions of solid in particular foods such as eggs and wheat which have a very high potential for sensitization.

In some infants, allergens from the mother may actually appear in the breast milk, thus sensitizing the baby.

Types of food allergy

The effects which food allergy may have on children remains a matter of some controversy. We will begin by describing those effects about which there is no disagreement, and then we will consider the more questionable aspects of the problem which relate to claims of food intolerance rather than to allergy.

Acute (type 1) reactions

Many individuals will have had at least one episode in which, apparently out of the blue, they develop severe abdominal cramp, with or without vomiting and diarrhoea, associated with a generalized itchy rash with wheals and urticaria (hives), swelling of the eyes or lips, and malaise which disappears as fast as it appears. The features, which are identical to some drug reactions, are almost certainly due to some food which is often unidentifiable. Occasionally it becomes obvious that a particular food is the offending agent because similar reactions occur whenever that food is eaten.

At the less severe end of the spectrum is the condition of recurrent urticaria (hives) which is a nuisance and not dangerous and may be a specific response to an easily identifiable food such as strawberries.

Acute reactions during infancy are most likely to be due to cows' milk or egg protein sensitivity. Obvious swelling, redness, or even blistering of the lips or skin round the mouth occurs on contact, followed by vomiting and diarrhoea. In the experience of the authors, egg is the most likely cause of this type of reaction but similar reactions may occur with cows' milk or wheat-containing foods.

At the extreme end of severity is the anaphylactic reaction with severe bronchospasm and circulatory failure. Some individuals develop swelling in the mouth immediately on contact with the food, and this may progress to oedema glottidis. Such extreme responses are fortunately rare. One of the author's brothers twice developed oedema glottidis on contact with Brazil nuts as a child yet has no other allergic symptoms.

When acute reactions occur with specific foods, avoidance of that food is the obvious solution, but the lengths to which one would go must depend on the severity of the symptoms. An individual who gets a few hives from strawberries and who has passion for the fruit might well decide the transient discomfort is a small price to pay for the delight. On the other hand an individual who develops severe glottal oedema at the merest contact with Brazil nuts would have to avoid them at all costs. Acute reactions to cows' milk formula in babies are the most commonly encountered. If the allergy is restricted to this then the use of a soya formula seems rational. Before making a change it is important to demonstrate by challenge that the reaction is indeed due to the formula. If the reaction is part of a wider picture of gastro-intestinal intolerance a more radical dietary approach is indicated (see below).

Eczema

Although eczema may appear at any age, it is the commonest form of allergy during infancy and can begin in very early life (under 6 weeks). It is important to distinguish between cradle cap with seborrhoeic dermatitis, which is usually a very transient condition and clears up after a few weeks and true infantile eczema. In some cases, apparent seborrhoeic dermatitis may progress to true infantile eczema. Both seborrhoea and eczema tend to begin on the face, but in true eczema, cracking of the skin particularly at the base of the ears becomes apparent and the rash spreads to the inner aspects of the elbows and knees and in severe cases becomes generalized. Sometimes, confusion may be caused by a severe form of nappy rash called psoriasiform dermatitis which has nothing to do with true atopy but may spread all over the body and can be cured with an application containing a fungicide, steroid, and antiseptic. It is important not to ascribe this condition to the infant's diet as this will lead to delay in effective treatment.

Infantile eczema may be very mild and may clear up very quickly. Nevertheless it is indicative of atopy and so could be a harbinger of more significant allergic states such as asthma later on in life.

DIAGNOSING FOOD ALLERGIES

Of the limited number of tests available which have some validity to confirm the presence of food allergy, skin tests and tests for

IgE (RAST tests) are the most commonly used. A strongly positive RAST to a particular food might argue against its attempted re-introduction, and we have on many occasions been able to re-introduce foods safely on the basis of negative results. Their value is however limited by lack of specificity and sensitivity. Detailed discussion of the indications and limitations of these methods is outside the scope of this text.

Many parents become obsessed with food allergy and try to seek help from sources where dubious diagnostic techniques, such as inadequately conducted provocation tests, hair analysis, and pulse testing, are employed. As a consequence they may be advised to place their children on diets which are unsound. We have come across several children who have been advised to avoid a wide variety of foods by so-called allergy clinics without being given necessary vitamin and mineral supplements and without proper assessment of energy needs. Parents have often paid large sums of money for tests and diet sheets of very poor quality which are both unhelpful and prone to errors. It can be very difficult to persuade these parents that after all their child is not allergic to foods and that they should revert to a normal diet.

Food challenges

Food challenges may be used in the initial diagnosis of food allergy and intolerance, or to confirm the diagnosis after a period of time on an exclusion diet. In most cases it is milk and dairy products which have been incriminated or excluded from the diet therefore the milk challenge is most widely used.

The introduction of milk to a child who has been on a milk-free diet for milk-protein intolerance or secondary lactose intolerance should not take place until a careful challenge has been carried out. The child is given a small quantity of milk while under medical supervision and if no reaction occurs, larger volumes are given at regular intervals over a few days. The exact method varies from centre to centre. If a reaction occurs, the diet should be resumed and the child re-challenged at some future date. If there is no reaction, a normal diet containing milk should be followed. Similar challenges can be carried out with other foods. In children who have previously had violent reactions to the food being re-introduced, the challenge should be carried out in hospital and adrenalin for immediate injection should be available.

Not infrequently a child may have inadvertently been exposed to milk or other excluded foods without developing a reaction. A careful dietary history may reveal that the child has been getting supposedly excluded foods in small quantities as ingredients in manufactured products. In these circumstances, the gradual re-introduction of milk or the excluded food should take place without a formal challenge.

In many situations the ideal test is to carry out a double-blind food challenge. This is particularly true where the effects are subjective or it is suspected that symptoms are being exaggerated or simulated. Blind challenges can be useful in convincing anxious parents that their child does not have a food allergy. Unfortunately they are difficult to perform because of the characteristic textures, tastes, and smells of foods. In genuinely doubtful cases they should be used despite these technical difficulties. Neither the parents, child, or person administering the food should be aware of what is being ingested. If the food can be powdered and given in a capsule or disguised in a 'safe' food, the procedure is simple. It is quite easy to hide tartrazine or other food colourings. It is much more difficult to disguise meat or fish or in situations where the symptoms are triggered by large quantities of food, i.e. migraine.

Exclusion diets, linked with challenges, if properly carried out, are helpful in diagnosing food allergy. The child is started on the diet for a period of time. If the symptoms improve, then other foods are gradually introduced. If the symptom recurs when a particular food has been re-introduced, then the offending food has been identified.

DIETARY TREATMENT OF FOOD ALLERGY

With all forms of suspected food allergy or food intolerance it is important that not only is a correct diagnosis made but that careful dietary advice is given. As we have stressed in other sections of this book, children have constantly changing dietary needs and it is essential that any special diet should take this underlying progression into account and be modified with time. The elimination of food from the diet will vary in each individual child with respect to the number of foods to be excluded and how strict an exclusion is necessary. The types of food excluded may vary according to the condition being treated. Some foods are known to cause problems in some situations but not in others.

It is crucially important to try to prevent parents seeking assistance from sources where there may not be a proper understanding of the nutritional needs of growing children. Such children may be exposed to a considerable risk of dietary deficiency with unconventional diets. There is also the added problem that apparent food allergy is yet another way in which Munchausen-by-proxy syndrome may present. Children who have no real allergy at all or only mild intolerance may have their symptoms exaggerated or fabricated.

There is evidence that children whose parents perceive that they are food allergic grow less well than other children. This may well be due not so much to the effects of allergy but to the long-term dietary imbalance which results from removing such items as milk, dairy products, and wheat from the diet without adequate nutritional advice. This is not to say that diet has no role to play in treating allergy, but that it should only be used where full evaluation has been carried out of the child and when dietetic expertise is available.

Exclusion diets

Exclusion diets may be used for the treatment of various forms of food allergy and intolerance, including eczema. The simplest form of exclusion or elimination diet is to remove one or two foods from the diet. This can usually only be done when there is a strong suspicion that the food is the one causing the problem, for example where symptoms are worse after the child consumes cows' milk.

The first step in deciding which foods are to be excluded is to ask the family to make a record of all the foods the child eats and to note down any reactions or worsening of symptoms. This can sometimes give a clue as to which foods should be excluded and a diet based on this information should be tried for one to four weeks.

Another alternative is to exclude several foods which are known to be likely causes of food allergy, for example milk, wheat, and eggs. The selection of foods may vary according to the condition. The advantage of the two above methods is that they involve minimal restriction of foods, which tends be easier for the family to follow. They do not, however, always provide an early answer since the foods causing the problem will not necessarily have been excluded. If there is no strong suspicion as to which food or foods the child cannot tolerate, a 'full exclusion' ('oligo-antigenic', 'oligo-allergenic' or 'few foods diet') is the most appropriate approach. These terms all describe a process whereby the diet is severely restricted to a few foods. The child's intake is limited to a small number of specified foods and usually includes one meat, a milk substitute, one vegetable or family of vegetables, one fruit, one cereal, a vegetable oil, and water. The diet also sometimes includes a margarine, sugar, and a low allergen drink such as colouring- and preservative-free lemonade.

Two examples of such diets are:

(1) turkey, cabbage, sprouts, broccoli, cauliflower, potato, banana, soya oil, water, and salt;

(2) lamb, carrots, parsnips, rice, pears, sunflower oil, water, and salt.

Both diets are deficient and require vitamin and mineral supplementation, and should on no account be used without dietary supervision.

These diets are complicated, expensive, and extremely difficult to follow, and in some cases may need to be started whilst the child is in hospital. It is usually recommended that the diet be followed for one to four weeks (Fig. 5.1). If the child's symptoms disappear, then the diet should continue and a gradual

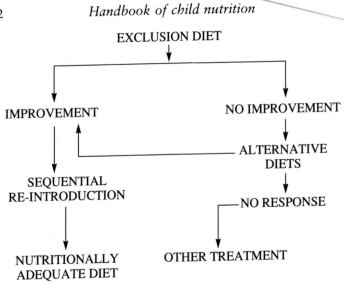

Fig. 5.1. Schema for exclusion diets.

re-introduction of other foods can commence. If the child does not respond, one must assume that food allergy or intolerance is not the diagnosis or that one of the foods allowed is the culprit, in which case a period of elemental diet or total parenteral nutrition may be considered in very severely affected children. In our experience this is very rarely indicated.

Exclusion diets in children require careful planning by an experienced dietitian working within a team framework in an experienced paediatric unit. The full co-operation of the parents and child is fundamental. The diets are not nutritionally adequate and require vitamin and mineral supplements. It may also be difficult to get the child to consume adequate energy, an important reason that the diet should only be followed for a short period of time.

Food re-introduction should take place carefully and systematically. In some clinics new foods are added every two days; in others once a week. The timing will depend on the likelihood of an acute reaction. The re-introduction requires careful dietetic supervision, otherwise confusion may easily arise. The food re-introduction need not follow a specific order but it seems sensible first to re-introduce foods least likely to cause a reaction. This quickly allows the diet to become more varied and nutritionally complete. Accurate records of food intake are necessary throughout this phase and it may take six months or even a year to complete the re-introduction fully.

It is obvious that full-scale exclusion diets are major undertakings fraught with potential hazard, and they should be reserved for those cases where the degree of ill-health caused by the allergy is of the first magnitude.

Diet in eczema

Food has been implicated as a cause of infantile and childhood eczema and this has led to two important views of management.

In the first place it is suggested that cows' milk protein is an important cause of eczema. Since almost all bottle-fed babies are fed formulas based on cows' milk it is inevitable that most babies who develop eczema will have been fed cows' milk, and this leads to the seemingly inevitable conclusion that cows' milk is the cause of the condition and that by avoiding it the risk of developing eczema will be reduced.

One obvious way of achieving this is exclusive breast-feeding. The other is to feed the baby with a formula based on a different source of protein i.e. soya. Unfortunately studies which have been done to attempt to determine whether soya is less likely to cause eczema have found no evidence of benefit. It may well be that the highly modified cows' milk-based formulas have proteins so denatured by the processes in their manufacture that they are no more likely to cause sensitization than soya. In fact the more that soya is used the more evident it becomes that it can also cause sensitization. There is at present no evidence to suggest that feeding potentially allergic babies soya rather than cows' milk based formulas has any benefit. The practice of starting potentially allergic babies on soya formula from birth is to be deprecated. If the baby has very severe eczema and if there is a family history of eczema which responded to food restriction, then the use of an elemental formula, under medical supervision, should be considered. There is insufficient evidence to justify providing elemental formulas on prescription in an attempt to prevent eczema or for eczematous children who do not have proven milk allergy.

Children from allergic families not already eczematous should be weaned in the normal way, but it may be prudent to avoid eggs and raw cows' milk until after the first year. Whether wheat should also be avoided is not certain unless the child is demonstrably sensitive to wheat.

The second view of management is that elimination diets may be of benefit to children who have already developed eczema. There are certainly some cases in which it is obvious that the ingestion of a particular food leads to an immediate flare up of the rash. Foods containing wheat, eggs, and milk have been especially associated with this type of reaction. In children in which this is so, it makes practical good sense to avoid the food or foods.

The trouble is that eczema is such a fluctuating condition and in many children there is a tendency to spontaneous remission with time. Psychological factors play a very important part in both the child and parents' perception of the severity of the symptoms. A state that is acceptable when all else is well can become intolerable during periods of stress.

It is against such a varying background that claims of benefit from diet manipulation have to be measured. There is at present no consensus as to the benefit of elimination diets in treating eczema. Opinion ranges from those who believe that dietary treatment is a complete waste of time and represents an example of the cure being worse than the disease, to those who would place all eczematous children on strict exclusion diets. Our view is that a strict exclusion diet may be of benefit to a very few children with intolerable symptoms which have not responded to conventional therapy, and whose lives are being made so miserable by their eczema that both they and their parents are willing to put up with the considerable difficulties of an oligo-antigenic diet regime. If this treatment is to be considered it is important that there is full co-operation from the child and parents and that adequate support is provided by medical and dietetic staff.

SPECIFIC GASTRO-INTESTINAL FOOD ALLERGY OR INTOLERANCE

Two specific forms of food intolerance are very important because they constitute potentially serious, even dangerous diseases. These are gastro-intestinal cows' milk protein intolerance and coeliac disease (gluten enteropathy). Fortunately, there is evidence that both conditions are on the wane, having reached a peak during the 1960s. Several reasons may account for this reduction in frequency. There seems little doubt that the new highly modified infant formulas are less likely to cause cows' milk sensitization than the old modified feeds. The fact that some 60–70 per cent of babies now receive some colostrum in early infancy is probably a contributing factor, and the increase in the proportion of babies being breast-fed for longer may be another factor. Additionally, there has been a significant fall in the incidence of gastro-enteritis in early infancy. Fewer babies thus sustain gastro-intestinal mucosal damage in early life and this may have some effect on reducing the risk of sensitization both to cows' milk protein and to gluten. Since the middle of the 1970s there has also been a significant reduction in the number of babies given gluten-containing foods in the first weeks of life, partly because the early introduction of solids has fallen sharply and partly because gluten-free cereals are now more widely used.

Cows' milk protein intolerance (gastro-intestinal)

This condition is characterized by vomiting and diarrhoea with failure to thrive, beginning at around six to eight weeks of life, although milder cases may occur later. Acute reactions which may be life threatening are seen in the more severe cases. Biopsy of the jejunum shows partial atrophy of the villi. The removal of cows' milk protein from the diet will lead to immediate and dramatic improvement. There has been some controversy as to whether these very ill babies should be fed soya formula such as Wysoy (Wyeth), Formula S (Cow & Gate), or Ostersoy (Farleys), or one of the elemental formulas, for example Pregestimil (Mead Johnson) or Pepti Junior (Cow & Gate). We recommend the latter despite the greater cost since there is a significant risk of soya intolerance developing in these infants.

A milk-free diet involves avoidance of all cows' milk products including butter, cheese, yoghurt, and cream. It is also necessary to exclude processed foods which contain milk products or milk derivatives including casein, whey, hydrolysed whey, and non-fat milk solids. These principles also apply during weaning, and care must be taken to check the ingredients listed on proprietary baby foods.

Some people suggest using goats' or ewes' milk instead of cows' milk for children with cows' milk intolerance. Under no circumstances should they be used as infant formula; in older children they may be used as a drink but there is a risk of intolerance developing to them as well. There is no evidence that milk from goats or sheep are less allergenic than that from cows. These milks must be purchased from a reliable source, and preferably should be pasteurized. Like cows' milk they contain lactose.

Some authorities recommend that once the child has regained weight and is well, a challenge with cows' milk should be carried out. It is characteristic of this condition that the milk intolerance disappears after infancy, usually at about 2 years of age, so that gradual re-introduction of milk-containing foods and eventually milk itself should be attempted at about this age. The initial challenge should be carried out under medical supervision because of the risk of an acute anaphylactic reaction in a very small number of children.

Coeliac disease (gluten enteropathy)

Coeliac disease is a disease of the proximal small intestine characterized by an abnormal mucosa and is associated with a permanent intolerance to gluten. It is due to sensitization to the protein gliadin, which is a component of gluten. The removal of gluten, which is present mainly in wheat, from the diet leads to a full clinical and pathological remission.

Recently the number of children diagnosed with coeliac disease has decreased. It is not known whether this is a true reduction of incidence or simply a delay in onset and diagnosis. It may be related to the fact that since the mid 1970s there has been a reduction in the very early introduction of solids of any kind and to the now common practice of delaying the introduction of wheat-containing cereals in the first months of life.

Children with coeliac disease may present in a variety of ways which include failure to gain weight or weight loss; anorexia; pale, soft, bulky, frequent stools; and irritability. The classical presentation of an intensely miserable, emaciated, and pot-bellied child was so characteristic that experienced paediatricians could diagnose the condition at a glance. Some cases may present with constipation whereas less severe cases of possibly later onset may present with short stature and/or anaemia.

The criteria for diagnosis are an abnormal small intestinal mucosa showing marked villous atrophy with a rapid clinical and histological response to dietary treatment.

The diet requires the exclusion of all gluten and gluten-containing products for life. Gluten is found in wheat, rye, barley, and oats. Some controversy exists as to whether it is necessary to exclude barley and oats since these cereals contain proteins which are slightly different to the gliadin found in wheat gluten. There have been varying reports on the effect they have on the intestinal mucosa, and in the light of recent research it is generally considered safer to exclude them from the diet.

The diet should be based on foods known to be gluten free including meat, fish, eggs, cheese, milk, vegetables, and fruits. Many manufactured products contain gluten and care must be taken to make sure products are gluten free; it is not always immediately apparent from the label. The Coeliac Society produces a list of manufactured foods free from gluten and the gluten-free symbol (see Fig. 5.2) can be seen on some products, particularly baby foods. There are a wide variety of special gluten-free products available, some on prescription. These include gluten-free flour, bread, biscuits, and cakes. These products are not necessarily low in protein since eggs and milk may have been used in their preparation. The inclusion of a wide

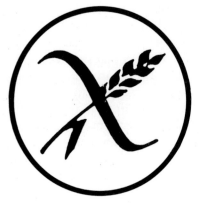

Fig. 5.2. The symbol of the Coeliac Society.

variety of gluten-free foods in the diet will ensure a nutritionally balanced diet and the child will grow at a normal rate.

The response to treatment in a classic case may be very dramatic (Fig. 5.3) but unfortunately as the child becomes older
compliance with diet may be less than good. This may have
potentially serious long-term consequences so it is very important
that individuals with proven coeliac disease should continue to
attend hospital clinics.

True coeliac disease is a permanent state and requires the
individual to remain on a gluten-free diet for life. There is,
however, a transient form of gluten enteropathy of infancy, and
therefore children at about 4 years of age should be given a
gluten challenge to see if symptoms recur. Repeat biopsy should
be carried out and if villous atrophy is present the child should
remain on a gluten-free diet for life. This challenge may be done
by giving the child gluten-containing foods such as bread and
biscuits, or by administering a gluten-containing powder. If the
dietary approach is used it is important to ensure that the child
actually ingests an adequate amount of gluten. If the child is no
longer gluten sensitive, the diet may be stopped. As with any
condition which damages the small intestinal wall, secondary
lactose intolerance may be present in untreated coeliacs, who
may well require a period on a lactose-free diet in addition.

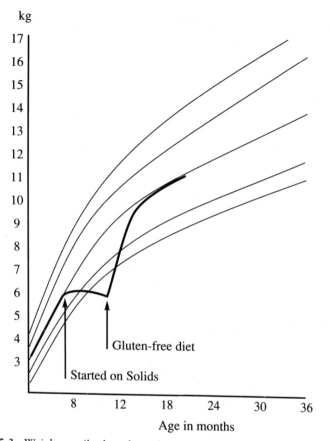

Fig. 5.3. Weight centile chart for girls aged 0–3 years showing response of child with coeliac disease to a gluten-free diet.

NON-ALLERGIC FOOD INTOLERANCE

Food intolerance not mediated by some disturbance of the immune mechanism may be due to untoward metabolic responses to food. There are some undoubted examples of this, such as enzyme defects, pharmacological reactions, or irritant effects, but also a great deal of controversy. Of course in many inborn errors of metabolism there are specific intolerances to particular molecules, i.e. phenylalanine in phenylketonuria or galactose in galactosaemia. These will be discussed in Chapter 9. However, some claims of harmful effects of certain foods and their components remain unproven.

Lactose intolerance

Lactose is the carbohydrate present in all mammalian milks. Lactose intolerance results from a deficiency of the enzyme lactase which is normally present in the brush borders of the mucous membranes of the jejunum. The symptoms of lactose intolerance are diarrhoea and failure to thrive, with foamy, acid stools and the presence of lactose in the stool, which is detected as a reducing substance to a test such as Clinitest.

Lactose intolerance may be a primary condition present at birth (primary alactasia) which is very rare and would be incompatible with prolonged survival unless the infant was placed on a lactose-free formula. Secondary lactose intolerance is much more common and is seen in all conditions where there is damage to the intestinal mucosa. Thus it may occur with or following such diseases as gastro-enteritis, coeliac disease or cows' milk protein intolerance. In these conditions it is transient. Treatment consists of avoiding lactose-containing foods until the bowel has recovered its lactase activity. Soya infant formulas contain no lactose and are suitable for this purpose provided the rest of the diet is lactose free. This is in all respects similar to a milk-free diet but some fermented products such as certain cheeses may in fact be lactose free and could be included in the diet. It is important to remember that some drugs and products such as toothpaste may contain lactose.

Another and most interesting form of lactose intolerance is seen in most racial groups other than Caucasians. This is the gradual disappearance of lactase activity from the bowel mucosa during later childhood so that in many peoples a proportion of the population is lactose-intolerant by adolescence, particularly males. On ingestion of raw milk, abdominal distension, pain, and diarrhoea occurs and these individuals quickly learn to avoid or limit milk or to ingest it only in a fermented form where the lactose has been converted to lactic acid. The nutritional importance of this phenomenon is that raw milk might not be a suitable dietary supplement for these older children and adolescents, and that they might consequently become calcium deficient. Many Afro-Caribbean and Asian children will become lactose intolerant as they get older.

Migraine

Migraine is one of those states in which the symptoms—visual aura, headache, nausea, vomiting, and abdominal pain—are the end point of a number of different factors in an individual with (probably inherited) predisposition. One factor (but not usually the most important) is intolerance to certain foods. Since there are many other factors which may precipitate an attack (see Fig. 5.4) and since in some migraine sufferers food does not appear to be a factor, the response to food avoidance is very variable and often disappointing. In some individuals where food is a factor, other factors are also present, so food avoidance may not stop attacks altogether.

The relative importance of the role of food intolerance in migraine remains controversial. Most authorities agree that certain amine-releasing foods, such as cheese, citrus fruits, and chocolate, may precipitate migraine attacks. Others would

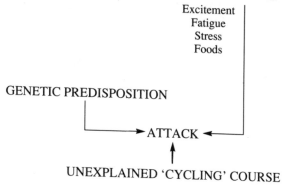

Fig. 5.4. Causes of migraine.

broaden the range of offending substances to include many common foods and food additives, notably tartrazine. Others have advocated an exclusion diet approach similar to that for allergic conditions. It is also suggested that hypoglycaemia may be a factor.

The exclusion-diet approach is not widely accepted for reasons which will be discussed in the next section.

Dietary management of migraine

In children with severe or frequent migraine, it is always worth considering a dietary approach to their treatment. This food avoidance approach is not difficult to enforce. In the light of our experience, the first approach should be to assess the child's overall nutritional intake and to ensure that a well-balanced diet is being eaten, with regular meals to avoid the possibility of hypoglycaemia. This is a simple approach requiring only a few dietary changes. The next step is the elimination of those foods from the diet which may have high vasoactive amine activity. These include such foods as cheese, chocolate, and game (Table 5.1).

Vasoactive agents are generally found in highest concentration in those foods which have undergone some decomposition or bacterial fermentation during their processing. Amino acids are converted into amines which are the active factors. They have long been suspected as being causes of migraine. Many adults and children will show reduction in number and severity of attacks if foods rich in vasoactive amines are removed from the diet. Foods with a high content of caffeine may also precipi-

Table 5.1. Foods high in vasoactive amines

Chocolate	Cheese
Yoghurt	Citrus fruits and juices
Banana	Pineapple
Raspberries	Plums
Peas	Broad beans
Avocado pear	Yeast and meat extracts
Shellfish	Smoked and pickled fish
Game	

tate migraine symptoms, and it may be sensible to avoid coffee, strong tea, and cola drinks.

The diet should be adhered to for two months and should become permanent if migraine attacks cease or become less frequent. Sequential re-introduction of the eliminated foods may be attempted but it may well be that it is the amount of vaso-active amine released overall rather than the effects of specific foods which is at fault. Thus foods taken in moderation may not cause an attack whereas a binge of, for example, chocolate ingestion will exact swift retribution. Many migraine sufferers will learn for themselves what degree of avoidance is needed to keep life tolerable.

If this approach is not successful it may be appropriate to exclude other foods, particularly if any are suspected of causing attacks. In severe cases of migraine an exclusion diet may determine whether foods cause a migraine attack. A diet similar to the one discussed earlier is usually used, and requires careful planning and monitoring by an experienced dietitian.

Such elaborate dietary regimes are rarely worthwhile and we would not recommend them in the routine treatment of migraine. Migraine is usually an intermittent state whereas the diet imposes continuous strain on child and family.

FOOD INTOLERANCE IN LESS WELL-DEFINED SITUATIONS

Food and food additives have been blamed for a wide range of symptoms in infants and chldren. 'Clinical ecologists' and 'allergy specialists', many using unconventional methods of diagnosis and treatment, are ready to diagnose food allergy much more readily than others. Doctors and other health professionals are often accused of being excessively sceptical about these claims and there are repeated demands from pressure groups for more allergy treatment and diagnosis to be available within the health service.

The reasons for the scepticism are both many and well-founded. Most important is the fact that the claims are often based on very poor scientific foundations. Dubious investigative procedures claiming to identify the presence of allergy by, for example, hair analysis abound. The clinical methods employed are themselves often very suspect and advocates fail to publish their results in a way capable of proper evaluation. On these grounds alone there must be a serious question mark over the validity of the claims, but more important the justification for demands for allocation of resources to procedures based on such unsound foundations requires very careful scrutiny.

A second ground for scepticism lies in the non-specific nature of the symptoms, the fact that they are often self-limiting and are open to other explanations. For example, hyperactivity in a 4 year old may be ascribed to, among other things, normal behaviour in a bright child whose parents for whatever reason find it difficult to cope with; imprudent rearing practices in which the child has not been properly disciplined to accept limits to acceptable behaviour; mental or neurological handicap due to pre-natal factors; and lack of stimulation or neglect. All these explanations are in varying degrees unwelcome and un-palatable, and it is all too easy to blame the child's behaviour on food additives or allergy. Subjecting such a child to complex diets may aggravate the problem and lead to failure to make the correct diagnosis.

Misdiagnosis is the third important reason for healthy scepticism in this field. Particularly during infancy, the risk of missing an important, treatable condition because of a wrong diagnosis of food allergy or intolerance is considerable. The authors have seen a number of such cases (see Table 4.2). It is obvious that errors of this type are potentially dangerous.

The fourth reason for scepticism is that the symptoms ascribed to food intolerance are in themselves often not a serious threat to long-term health, and thus the 'cure'—elaborate dieting —may be worse than the 'disease', partly because of the major inconvenience to all concerned, the not inconsiderable nutritional risks, and the psychological effects of 'labelling' children with a doubtful diagnosis. The best example of this is the condition 'toddler diarrhoea' which is discussed elsewhere in detail.

'Hyperactivity'

Since this is the most notorious example of what is usually a behaviour disturbance being ascribed to food intolerance, it deserves a section on its own. The facts are that most children diagnosed as 'hyperactive' are perfectly normal children bouncing with undirected energy. Thus most children being placed on diets for hyperactivity are either perfectly normal or have other explanations for their behaviour. Furthermore the evidence that there is a sub-group of hyperactive children who might benefit from additive-free diets remains very dubious. Independent double-blind studies have failed to reveal benefit, and anecdotal claims of response in individual children are open to all the usual criticisms in situations where there are often powerful psychological factors at work and where the symptoms are likely to resolve with time anyway.

Health-care workers find themselves in some difficulties in this and similar situations. Many parents have become thoroughly convinced that the diet is to blame for their children's problems. The media have lost no opportunity to use this issue to play their familiar game of bashing the 'Establishment'. Some reporters seem quite extraordinarily gullible in their eager willingness to believe the most ludicrous notions. Advocates of 'unconventional methods' feel none of the inhibitions against outrageous public pronouncements and totally unsubstantiated claims which make headlines and which are so difficult to counter.

Many children, as in the case of those being treated for allergy, are put onto diets on the advice of 'self-help' groups or professionals with little knowledge or understanding of children's nutritional needs. Since many of the 'conditions' being treated are not organic or are self-limited, or are in the minds of the parents rather than the bodies of their children, it is not difficult for such practitioners or their dubious methods to chalk up 'successes' when all others have 'failed' or have 'refused to recognize the true nature' of the complaint. This is a growing and worrying problem for which there is no obvious immediate solution. Health workers are on a hiding to nothing in attempting to deal with such cases. If they refuse to become involved, the child may suffer serious nutritional harm. If they assist the parents to maintain diets for non-existent diseases, they are perpetuating the evil. When such families are encountered, there is a responsibility to help the parents to find a rational solution to their children's difficulties, or at the very least to ensure that their diets are adequate.

Although there is no strong evidence to implicate artificial colouring agents and other additives, there is no reason why processed foods which contain them should not be eliminated from the diet. Not all so-called E-numbers are artificial agents, and many have been included in foods from time immemorial. The E-numbers are a list of food additives generally regarded as safe for use within the European Community. They include naturally occurring colourants, gums, vitamins, and preservatives. Examples of these are given in Table 5.2. There are certain groups of E-numbers, particularly artificial colours and preservatives, which may be suspect and are probably well avoided. These include the well-known colouring agents E102 (tartrazine) and E110 (sunset yellow). Both are azo dyes. Preservatives include the benzoate group E210–219. Both the azo dyes and benzoates have been known to cause asthmatic attacks in susceptible individuals. Their implications on behaviour is less well documented. They are, however, fairly easy to avoid and

Table 5.2. Examples of natural permitted additives

Colours	
Caramel (brown)	E150
Riboflavin (yellow)	E101
Chlorophyl (green)	E140
Carbon (black)	E153
Alpha carotene (Yellow, orange)	E160 (a)
Preservative	
Acetic acid	E260
Lactic acid	E270
Anti-oxidants	
Ascorbic acid and derivatives	E300–305
Tocopherols	E306–309
Emulsifiers and stabilizers	
Citric acid and its derivatives	E330–333
Agar	E406
Pectin	E440

unnecessary additions to the diet. A diet based largely on fresh, unprocessed foods is more likely to meet healthy eating recommendations.

DIETARY SUGAR AND BEHAVIOUR PROBLEMS

Some writers have claimed that an increased intake of sucrose may cause learning and behaviour difficulties in schoolchildren (see Chapter 9).

ALUMINIUM IN INFANT FEEDS

Concern has recently been expressed regarding the very high aluminium levels found in some baby foods, particularly soya and special formulas. The more manipulation the food undergoes, the higher the aluminium content is likely to be. Although there is no objective evidence that even the very high levels which have been detected in soya formulas are actually harmful, worry is understandable in view of the tentative but still unproven links which have been made between aluminium intake and various degenerative conditions. Our view is that the new observations give further strength to the argument that soya formulas and other special feeds should not be used for treating trivial and self-limiting conditions such as colic. Nor should they be given to babies with unsubstantiated 'cows milk intolerance' or in the unjustified hope that allergy may be prevented. In those conditions where the well-being of the infant depends on the use of soya or other special formulas, they should continue to be used.

6

The preschoolchild

It is a remarkable fact that whereas much is known about the diets of sucklings and weanlings as a result of the excellent surveys carried out by the Office of Population Censuses and Surveys (OPCS) and also about the diets of schoolchildren, there is little useful information about what toddlers and preschool-children eat, although there are clearly defined recommendations (Table 6.1). Few studies in Britain have examined the diets of children between 1 and 5 years of age. In the United States, at least one study (Bogalusa) indicates that preschoolchildren have high energy intakes comprised of a large proportion of refined sugar and saturated fat. If British figures are similar this would be a cause for great concern.

Questions remain unanswered as to the amounts of fat, fibre, and overall energy that children in this age group require or can tolerate. This information is likely to be difficult to obtain, yet without it, it is not possible to start to form a rational policy for advice on eating because this might be unrelated to what most children eat and therefore unlikely to be successful. Nevertheless some policy has to be evolved in the interim.

The problems of encouraging a healthy diet have been discussed in Chapter 2, and current opinion favours a gradual rather than sudden increase in fibre and reduction of fats from the amounts ingested during infancy.

There are certain specific nutritionally related problems which occur in otherwise normal children, are not manifestations of serious illness, and are self-limiting, but nevertheless are a serious cause of inconvenience and parental anxiety. These conditions include eating difficulties, toddler diarrhoea, and constipation.

Table 6.1 Recommended daily intakes of energy and nutrients for children aged 1 to 18 years

Age (years)	Weight (kg)	Energy (kcal)	Protein (g)	Vitamins						Minerals	
				Thiamin (mg)	Riboflavin (mg)	Nicotinic acid (mg equiv.)	C (mg)	A (μg^1)	D^2 (g)	Calcium (mg)	Iron (mg)
1–2³	11.4	1200	30	0.5	0.6	7	20	300	10	500	7
2–3³	13.5	1400	35	0.6	0.7	8	20	300	10	500	7
3–5³	16.5	1600	40	0.6	0.8	9	20	300	10	500	8
5–7³	20.5	1800	45	0.7	1.0	10	20	300	2.5	500	8
7–9³	25.1	2100	53	0.8	1.0	11	20	400	2.5	500	10
Boys											
9–12	31.9	2500	63	1.0	1.2	14	25	575	2.5	700	13
12–15	45.5	2800	70	1.1	1.4	16	25	725	2.5	700	14
15–18	61.0	3000	75	1.2	1.7	19	30	750	2.5	600	15
Girls											
9–12	33.0	2300	58	0.9	1.2	13	25	575	2.5	700	13
12–15	48.6	2300	58	0.9	1.4	16	25	725	2.5	700	14
15–18	56.1	2300	58	0.9	1.4	16	30	750	2.5	600	15

Taken from DHSS No 120 Recommended Daily Intakes of Nutrients for the United Kingdom.
[1] Retinol equivalent.
[2] Cholecalciferol.
[3] Boys and girls.

A BALANCED DIET FOR THE TODDLER

There are several stages in the feeding development of the pre-schoolchild, from messy finger-feeding at one year to becoming a competent eater using child-sized cutlery at 4–5 years of age. The intermediate stages include the spoon and bowl used by the 2 year old and the spoon, fork, and plate wielding 3 year old.

What should toddlers be eating? Many people believe that it is important to establish good eating patterns from early childhood since this is likely to establish 'healthy' nutritional patterns for life. Whether there is justification for such a view remains uncertain, but on basic principles, the proposition appears sensible. Many British children have extraordinarily unvaried diets and it is possible that this might make them prey to badly balanced food intakes later in life.

Toddlers are often 'faddy' eaters, which causes parents considerable anxiety and certainly makes it difficult to ensure that their children have a diet containing a variety of foods. Young children have small stomachs, small appetites, and may not be able to consume all they need without between-meal snacks which play an important part in their nutrition. Three meals plus two or three snacks should be offered, with a variety of foods of differing tastes, textures, and colours which will help maintain the child's interest.

Sugary and sweet foods should not form a major part of the diet, partly because they make the child reluctant to eat other foods and therefore a taste for variety is not developed, also they provide 'empty' calories requiring frequent intake to stave off hunger, and they will cause dental caries.

Examples of suitable snack meals for children of different ages are given in Table 2.4.

THE CHILD WHO 'WON'T EAT'

Many toddlers go through phases of food reluctance or food refusal. These may be due to 'fads' or be part of a strategy of attention seeking. In its less extreme form and when handled sensibly by parents this is part of normal maturation. In some situations where there is parental (not infrequently grandparental) overreaction, a vicious cycle of parental anxiety emerges. This leads to the child enjoying the advantages of greater attention, and results in further refusal to eat.

Transient refusal to eat may be associated with minor illnesses or emotional upsets such as the death of a pet. Children on very restrictive therapeutic diets may refuse to eat and in some circumstances this can lead to major difficulties.

Children are frequently brought to see doctors or other health workers with the complaint that they will not eat. Physical examination and recording the child's weight on a centile chart will usually reveal that there is no evidence of undernutrition. If this is the case, the first essential is to attempt to reassure the parents that there is nothing seriously wrong. This will not be achieved by multiple investigations or stray comments about possible food intolerance.

Food refusal and food fads (toddler strikes) are often part of an overall pattern of behaviour seen in toddlers, particularly at around 2 years of age, a period sometimes called the 'terrible twos'. In most cases the child is very well, or even over-nourished, and the problem may be the parent's perception of what they think the child should be eating. Some youngsters have learned to use meal-times as an excellent way to test out their parents, and refuse the food offered precisely because of the anxiety which it engenders. Occasionally the problem is a superficial manifestation of deeper-seated family difficulties which should be excluded. The occasional toddler goes on 'hunger-strike' as a form of attention seeking in response to a new sibling.

The child may become overtly manipulative and meals can turn into a battle of wills which the child is bound to win. All pleading will be in vain and force-feeding attempts will be utterly counter-productive. By the time the family is referred, the situation may have deteriorated to the point where meals have become a nightmare, family relationships have deteriorated, and considerable emotional distress engendered.

The first requirement in these situations is to establish that the child is not undernourished. Plotting height and weight on a centile chart and demonstrating them to the parents is usually sufficient to achieve this, but in some instances, particularly where milk is being rejected, a dietary assessment may be useful. If the child is thriving and there is no suggestion of any deficiencies, the parents should be reassured that their child is most unlikely to starve himself to death and that the best policy, easier to suggest than to carry out, is to ignore the whole matter. Food should be offered, the child given those that he or she likes, and if the meal is refused it should be removed after a reasonable period. Children, like adults, have food preferences. No attempt should be made either to entice or force the child to eat and no food should be offered until the next meal.

As long as the child continues to gain weight at a rate appropriate to its height, no further action is needed. If it is clear that the child is underweight or that the rate of gain is less than it should be, then the child should be referred to a paediatrician to exclude an organic cause. Even then it is likely that nothing significant will be found. Some otherwise healthy children are eating a less than optimal diet, often with an energy intake too low to secure optimal growth or with deficiencies of vitamins or minerals (particularly iron or calcium). In such cases some sort of dietary supplementation should be given and a careful record kept of height and weight. Dietetic advice is useful to ensure that the diet is not defective in some way and to suggest strategies to increase the intake. Quite minor dietary modification may resolve the problem. Parents become more relaxed about the food refusal and the child begins to eat normally. Encouraging the child to eat with its peer group at nursery and day-care centre may be helpful. In older children between 3–4 years of age, simple behaviour modification using star charts and a reward system is worth trying but it is important to include the dietitian, health visitor, or doctor in its implementation.

Provided there is no underlying organic disease, the problem always resolves eventually.

BIZARRE DIETS

Toddlers often restrict their intake to a very narrow range of foods, for example, diets consisting of milk, crisps, and bread only, or baked beans, and corn flakes. These bizarre diets will cause great worry to parents and health professionals. In fact such diets often contain much of what the child requires and attempts at forcing the child to eat anything else will not succeed. This pattern often lasts only for a few weeks, following which the child eats a different combination of foods. Over a period of time a series of diets not adequate in themselves will provide an overall balance. A variety of foods should always be offered and patience will eventually be rewarded. Occasionally the problem is due to the intake of huge volumes of milk which prevents the child taking other foods. Milk intake should be restricted to between one to two pints per day, allowing the child to eat other foods. Changing the child from a feeder to an ordinary cup can reduce the amount of fluid taken.

ARE SUPPLEMENTARY VITAMINS NECESSARY?

Most infants who are either breast-fed or fed a standard infant formula will at the time of weaning have had adequate intake of vitamins. The only doubts among normal full-term babies concerns ascorbic acid (vitamin C) because it is heat labile, and the fat-soluble vitamins A and D because they depend to some extent on the level of fat absorption, the presence of stores in the liver and fatty depots, and because the levels present in infant formula may be insufficient for the occasional baby. The ascorbic acid content of breast milk depends on maternal intake. Giving a standard vitamin drop preparation containing A, D, and C from about 6 weeks of age to all infants seems a reasonable precaution.

Once the child is weaned, the dietary content of these three vitamins will depend on the intake, which may be variable enough to cause problems. For example a child who does not like milk, fresh vegetables, or fruit might well develop deficiencies of ascorbic acid and/or fat-soluble vitamins. Adequacy of intake cannot be assured without detailed dietary assessment and for this reason supplementary vitamins A, D, and C are recommended until school age (see Table 1.4).

Some parents take exception to what they see as unnecessary dosing of their children with vitamins. Most nutritional authorities agree that provided energy and protein intake is adequate, deficiency is unlikely. Those parents who feel very strongly can be reassured that their children will not suffer, provided they have good dietary sources of vitamins.

On the other hand there are some parents who seem to become obsessed with the idea that their children are deficient in vitamins. There is no evidence that children on healthy diets or those receiving supplements as recommended are likely to suffer because they have inadequate vitamin intake and there is no case for additional administration. There is a risk that overdosage with fat-soluble vitamins in particular may result. We discuss the role of vitamins in the diets of infants in Chapter 1 and schoolchildren in Chapter 9.

TODDLER DIARRHOEA (NON-SPECIFIC DIARRHOEA)

This condition usually presents between 6 and 20 months of age and appears to coincide with the period of weaning onto solid foods and usually ceases by the third year of life. The symptoms are increased stool frequency, diarrhoea, and abdominal pain, but without growth problems. Undigested particles of food such as peas and carrots are seen in the stools. Characteristically the children remain very well and have good appetites.

Causes

There are several possible explanations for toddler diarrhoea. These include recurrent minor infections which the child picks up as a result of increased mobility. The reduction of fat intake associated with weaning is thought to be a factor, because reduced fat speeds up gastric emptying. If this trend is accelerated by placing the child on skimmed or semi-skimmed milk and adding excessive amounts of fibre to the diet in line with current notions on healthy eating, the 'muesli-belt' syndrome of chronic diarrhoea and undernutrition may result. Parents may become fanatical about their own diets and expect their children to follow suit.

Some workers have suggested that toddler diarrhoea may be due to food allergy. In our experience this is not the case and parents should not be encouraged to think that complex dietary manipulation will be beneficial. Here, as elsewhere, the casual suggestion that a child might have food intolerance can have serious consequences.

Children with toddler diarrhoea should not be over-investigated. If linear growth and weight gain is satisfactory and the child is otherwise well, further tests are not indicated apart from stool culture and checking for reducing substances.

Management

Management should begin with reassurance of the parents that there is nothing seriously wrong with the child and that the diarrhoea will eventually stop. This in itself will often suffice since parents will accept a transient nuisance if they know it is not dangerous. A brief dietary history will establish whether the diet contains excess fibre or inadequate fat, and it should be adjusted accordingly. If there is poor fat intake this may be because the child has stopped drinking milk or is given skimmed milk. The parents should be advised to increase the intake of whole milk to at least one pint per day. If the child does not like milk, flavourings can be tried to make milkshakes, or alternatives such as cheese and yoghurt may be given along with other foods which have a relatively high fat content (Fig. 6.1).

A diet which is too high in fibre will feature many wholegrain cereals, bran-supplemented foods and sometimes added bran. Pure bran should not generally be given to young children and its use should be stopped in any child with diarrhoea. Some reduction in the content of wholegrains may also be necessary. Curiously there is a view that toddler diarrhoea may be alleviated by increasing the dietary fibre, but we know of no convincing evidence to support this opinion.

Drug therapy to slow bowel movements has been advocated but it is our view that this is best avoided.

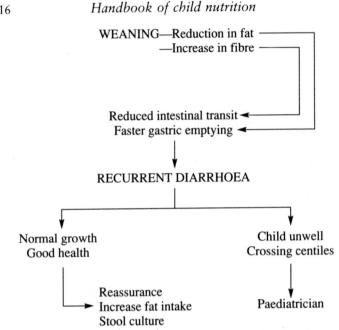

Fig. 6.1. Toddler diarrhoea.

In some children with toddler diarrhoea, establishing toilet training may alleviate symptoms.

CONSTIPATION

The problems associated with constipation tend to occur after attempts at toilet training. From about 2 years of age, faecal retention often associated with soiling becomes increasingly common. The cause of this distressing condition is complex. The principle of treatment we recommend is to ensure that the child evacuates the rectum at regular intervals. This prevents accumulation of faeces and the resultant secondary megacolon which it induces. Paradoxically one of the elements in this is to increase faecal bulk. Laxatives have their part to play, and opinions vary as to how large this should be and which laxative to use. They should not be seen as a long-term solution but as a stepping stone to the establishment of a normal bowel habit.

The general management of constipation in preschoolchildren

consists of a group of measures which include laxatives as a short-term measure, behaviour modification using star charts and positive re-inforcement, together with a high-fibre diet.

It would be a mistake to place too much reliance on diet alone in severe cases. No doubt, a general increase in fibre intake will reduce the prevalence of constipation, but those who have attempted to treat large numbers of severely constipated and soiling younger children will know that its role is at the best supportive. On the other hand, simple, less severe constipation will respond quite well to a high-fibre diet. There are two ways of achieving this.

1. Persuade the whole family to change their diet towards greater fibre intake. It is counter-productive for all the family members to tuck into slices of white bread while the child is left miserably contemplating a thick, to him, unappetizing lump of rough brown loaf. If the brown bread is so good, why is everybody not eating it?

2. A reasonable increase in fibre in the individual child is attained by mixing fibre-rich cereal with the child's own favourite breakfast food.

We have found the star chart approach used for our general management of constipation useful in achieving some increased intake in younger children. Stars are awarded each time the child eats a portion containing fibre.

This dietary programme is combined with behaviour modification directed towards achieving a regular bowel habit. The child is encouraged to sit on the toilet every day at a specific time and a star awarded for this. Additionally, stars are gained by successful defecation and absence of soiling. A contract is agreed whereby once the child has achieved an appropriate number of stars a reward will be given by one of the parents.

A major problem is that many of the families with children with truly resistant constipation and soiling, have major social and emotional problems. For them a radical dietary change only adds to their general burdens. These children tend to remain constipated for years and it is not clear what eventually happens to them.

THE HIGH-FIBRE DIET

Dietary fibre consists of non-starch polysaccharides which are complexes of cellulose. They are mainly derived from the cell walls of plants, and are generally passed through the intestine in an undigested form and are therefore not absorbed. The aim of a high-fibre diet is to include as many unrefined and fibrous foods as possible. This can be achieved in the following ways.

1. Eat more bread—especially wholemeal, granary, or high bran. For those who do not like these an alternative is high-fibre white bread.

2. Start the day with a cereal high in fibre such as Weetabix, Shredded Wheat, Shreddies, Puffed Wheat, All-bran, Bran Flakes, Sultana Bran, porridge, Weetaflakes and muesli (avoid cereals containing whole nuts in young children).

3. Eat more vegetables, including, peas, beans, lentils, and potatoes in their skins.

4. Eat plenty of fruit, including the skins. Dried fruits are particularly high in fibre.

5. Try wholemeal pasta and brown rice.

6. Use wholemeal flour in baking and purchase products containing wholemeal flour.

7. Drink plenty of fluid.

7

Diet and diarrhoea

DIARRHOEA in infants and young children is defined as the frequent passage of watery stools. Excessive loss of intestinal contents, acute or chronic, may have nutritional implications either because of the direct loss of nutrients, or because diarrhoea is a symptom of malabsorption.

ACUTE DIARRHOEA

Diarrhoea is described as acute when its onset is sudden and its duration is limited. The main risk to the child is dehydration, and the electrolyte disturbance associated with it. On a world-wide basis, diarrhoeal disease is second only to malnutrition as a cause of infant death. It is also a major factor in pushing children with borderline nutrition into full-blown protein-calorie malnutrition.

In developed countries, particularly with improvements in infant feeding, it has become a much less severe condition than in the past. Younger infants are at greater risk; they are more vulnerable to acute water loss because they have higher basal requirements and less robust compensatory renal mechanisms. They are also more likely to develop the complications of secondary mucosal damage leading to lactose and cows' milk or soya protein intolerance.

Breast-feeding provides protection against gastro-enteritis, partly because it contains no pathogens likely to cause diarrhoeal disease and partly because it provides antibacterial and viral agents which are protective. Furthermore it appears that babies who are breast-fed are less likely than artificially fed babies to develop dehydration or electrolyte disturbances. Bottle feeds and solid food can be contaminated with bacteria, particularly where there is lack of refrigeration, where hygienic conditions are not good and where the water supply is contaminated. In some parts of the world, bottle-feeding is almost certain to lead to diarrhoeal disease.

Causes

Most acute diarrhoea (gastro-enteritis) is infectious in origin. The causative organisms are commonly viral (rotavirus), but may be bacterial (salmonella, shigella, campylobacter) or protozoal (amoebiasis). The younger the child, the more likely it is that the cause will be viral because bacterial contamination of correctly prepared formula is rare. Bacterial gastro-enteritis can cause serious illness. There have been several recent disturbing episodes of salmonella contamination of infant formula and weaning food in the factories. In developing countries the problem is quite different because contamination of water supplies results in bacterial gastro-enteritis occurring in young infants who are formula fed.

Nutritional effects

Most acute diarrhoea in otherwise healthy children will not affect nutrition, but in malnourished children it can be a serious complication leading to a further deterioration of nutritional status. Young babies in particular, develop mucosal damage to the small bowel which may be more chronic. Children who have chronic diseases are likely to develop more serious nutritional problems.

Food intolerance, either primary or secondary to gastro-enteritis, is an important cause of persistent diarrhoea and is discussed in Chapter 5.

Management

Managing the child with acute diarrhoea involves two main objectives.

1. Prevention and treatment of dehydration with its associated electrolyte disturbance.
2. Maintenance or resumption of adequate nutrition.

It has become traditional to divide children with diarrhoea into three clinical categories, mild, moderate, and severe, based on the state of hydration. Mild dehydration corresponds to a loss of body weight of less than 5 per cent. Moderate dehydration describes those who have lost between 5 and 10 per cent body weight, while the severely dehydrated child has lost at least 10 per cent of its body weight. It is not the purpose of this book to describe in detail the treatment of diarrhoeal disease, but it seems appropriate to outline those aspects concerned with the administration of oral rehydration and nutrition (Fig. 7.1).

Mildly dehydrated children can usually be managed quite safely at home. It is usually prudent to provide a specially constituted water and electrolyte solution containing some glucose or other sugars which can be given to the child *ad libitum*.

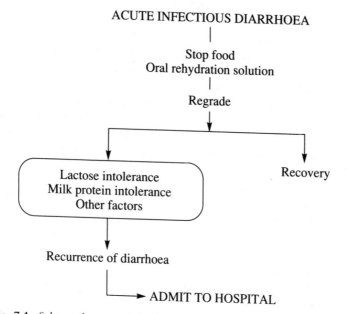

Fig. 7.1. Schema for acute infectious diarrhoea.

The various preparations available in this country and suitable for home therapy are listed in Table 7.1. Solutions containing higher concentrations of sodium such as the WHO oral rehydration fluid should be reserved for hospital treatment in developed countries and should not be given to parents to administer at home.

Whether ordinary feeding should continue or whether food should be stopped for a limited period to 'rest the bowel' has been a matter of recent controversy. Breast-fed babies should continue to be fed despite the theoretical risk that the baby might have secondary lactose intolerance. This has become so rare in this group of infants as to be of no real practical importance.

It is still customary in this country, in bottle-fed or weaned infants, to treat acute infectious diarrhoea with a period of starvation apart from the administration of an oral rehydration fluid, providing the infant is otherwise healthy and well nourished, following which most can be restarted on normal diet once the stools have abated.

Feeding should be re-established as soon as possible, and certainly no baby should be starved for more than 48 hours without seeking expert advice and probably admission to hospital. Traditionally there is a gradual introduction of milk, starting with a dilute formula and then progressively increasing both concentration and volume as the infant demonstrates tolerance. Whether this is necessary for mild diarrhoea in healthy infants is questionable but it is probably prudent to use it in more severe cases, particularly babies who have needed intravenous therapy. Malnourished babies have special problems which may require a different approach.

The aim of re-grading is to prevent dehydration by ensuring that at first a significant proportion of the intake is the oral rehydrating solution. It will also prevent explosive recurrence of diarrhoea if an intolerance has developed. In some babies mild, loose stools may persist for a few days even with this approach. If this becomes severe, the baby should be admitted without delay. A second period of starvation should not be undertaken at home.

Table 7.1. Some oral rehydration fluids suitable for home use

Solution (per 100ml)	Energy (kcal)	Carbohydrate (g)	Sodium (mmol)	Potassium (mmol)	Chloride (mmol)
Dextrolyte 100ml ready to feed	14	Glucose-3.6	3.5	1.3	3.0
Dioralyte 1 sachet in 200ml water	16	Glucose-4	3.5	2.0	3.7
Electrolade 1 sachet in 200ml water	9	Glucose-2.2	5.0	2.0	4.0
Electrosol 1 sachet in 200ml water	16	Glucose-4	3.5	2.0	3.7
Gluco-lyte 1 sachet in 200ml water	16	Glucose-4	3.5	2.0	3.7
Paedialyte MS 250ml ready to feed	11	Glucose-2.8	4.5	2.0	3.5
Rehidrat 1 sachet in 250ml water	15	Glucose Fructose-3.7 Sucrose	5.0	2.0	5.0

A typical re-grading programme over a period of two to four days is as follows:

1/4 strength formula + 3/4 oral rehydration fluid;
1/2 strength formula + 1/2 oral rehydration fluid;
3/4 strength formula + 1/4 oral rehydration fluid;
full strength formula.

The formula should be made up in the usual way with water and then diluted with oral rehydration fluid.

A similar procedure may be followed with the older child, using cows' milk and oral rehydration solution with a gradual re-introduction of solids. The great majority of children will accept re-grading with a cows'-milk based formula, and only a small number will require a special formula. For some reason, secondary lactose intolerance appears to have become much less common than in the past.

A special formula specifically designed for re-grading has recently been introduced. This product, HN25 (Milupa), contains protein, energy, vitamins, and minerals, but in lower concentrations than in normal formula. It has a higher concentration of sodium and potassium than ordinary formula, in order to meet the increased losses of diarrhoeal disease. It is classified as a low-lactose feed becuse it is not entirely lactose free, containing about 1/70th of the concentration of lactose in normal infant formula. This product is not a complete infant formula and is only suitable for use over a short period of time. It can be made up to a 'milk-like' feed with water, not oral rehydration fluid, or mixed to a paste as a solid food. There is a potential risk in mixing the powder with oral rehydration fluid as the solute load, particularly from the sodium, could be considerable. If used as a solid, care must be taken to ensure an adequate intake of fluid. The manufacturers claim, with some scientific support, that it can be used at full strength immediately following rehydration, and that it may shorten the recovery period, whilst giving improved nutrition. It is our opinion that this product is probably not necessary for most children with gastro-enteritis in Britain, who are generally well-nourished pror to the onset of their diarrhoea and who recover satisfactorily with the usual re-grading process. It may have a useful role in malnourished children. As it is not a complete infant feed it should only be used with appropriate medical and dietetic supervision.

Nutrition becomes a problem in those babies who are malnourished from the start, or in infants who have persisting diarrhoea after re-grading because they have developed transient lactose or milk protein intolerance. The stool should be tested for reducing substance and if present should be sent to the laboratory for chromatography to confirm that lactose is present.

Special formulas

If lactose intolerance is present then the baby should be tried on a soya-based infant formula which is lactose-free. Alternatively a hydrolysed whey or casein-based formula may be used e.g. Pregestimil (Mead Johnson), Nutramigen (Mead Johnson), and Pepti Junior (Cow & Gate). It is usually possible to re-introduce ordinary feeds within a week or two, once the baby has regained its previous weight.

If recurrent diarrhoea has occurred after re-grading without lactose in the stool, the possibility of transient milk-protein intolerance must be considered and, in view of the fact that at least some of these babies will become lactose intolerant as well, such infants should be placed on an hydrolysed formula for a few weeks with cautious re-introduction of a milk-based feed after challenge.

Admission to hospital

Although most diarrhoeal disease is mild and can be treated effectively at home, there should be no hesitation in admitting children, particularly infants, if there is any doubt. The following criteria may be helpful in deciding whether the child should be treated in hospital:

(1) poorly nourished children;

(2) recurrence of diarrhoea after regrading;

(3) persistence of diarrhoea despite period of starvation;

(4) vomiting of electrolyte solutions;

(5) dehydration in excess of 5 per cent or evidence of acidosis (rapid breathing);

(6) bloody diarrhoea;

(7) oliguria.

CHRONIC DIARRHOEA OTHER THAN TODDLER DIARRHOEA

There are some very rare and dangerous forms of persistent chronic diarrhoea of infancy which are intractable and which require highly specialized management. These conditions sometimes are preceded by gastro-enteritis (see Chapter 10).

'DIARRHOEA DE RETOUR'

Many parents who have recently migrated to Europe like to take their young children back to their homelands to be seen by relatives. The change in bacterial flora and food often causes diarrhoea which in severe cases may go on to cause malnutrition and persistent intractable diarrhoea on return to Britain. A similar condition was first described in France in children returning there from Algeria and Morocco. It is very important to recognize this entity early and not to attempt domiciliary treatment with starvation and re-grading as this will aggravate the situation. These children will often have developed secondary lactose intolerance, cows' milk or soya intolerance, and the problem may be complicated by worm infestation. They may have become infected by unusual bacterial organisms. These children require specialist management and the introduction of oral feeding can very difficult. A period of lactose-free feeding or even the use of an elemental formula may be appropriate. There should be very careful monitoring of nutritional status, and recurrence of diarrhoea must be regarded very seriously and may require parenteral nutrition.

DANGERS OF SPECULATIVE MANAGEMENT

All babies with significant persistent diarrhoea require expert attention. It is dangerous to assume diagnoses such as lactose intolerance and milk-protein intolerance without careful assessment.

8

Obesity

THE common-sense view is that people, including children, get fat because they eat too much. Yet there is important evidence that excessive food intake is not the only or necessarily the most important reason for childhood obesity. Genetic predisposition acting through a metabolic mechanism may account for the fact that some children get fat on diets not very different from those on which other children remain lean. Nevertheless, levels of energy intake which are generally increased are bound to lead to a greater prevalence of obesity. It is a truism that obesity is due to an excess energy intake over expenditure (Fig. 8.1).

PREVALENCE OF OBESITY

There are large differences in estimates of the prevalence of obesity in children. This may stem in part from differences in the type of measurement and criteria used for diagnosing obesity, although it is also obvious that there are genuine differences from country to country and among different ethnic groups and social classes. Such differences are not always consistent; in one society obesity may be a feature of the privileged, whereas in other societies it is seen predominantly in lower social strata. There may also be genuine ethnic variations in the genetic potential for adiposity.

Adult obesity is more common in the United States than elsewhere and childhood obesity is on the increase, with substantial increases in obesity detected between 1963 and 1980. Obesity may have increased by 54 per cent and 'super-obesity' by 98 per cent in children between 6 and 11 years, with similar changes in adolescents. It is also alarming that the fat children

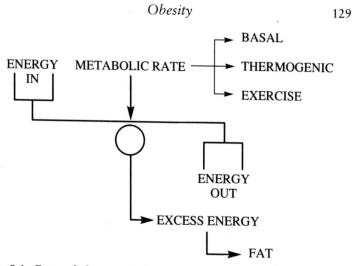

Fig. 8.1. Energy balance and obesity.

are more obese than they were previously. The lesson of these findings is that there are probably environmental factors at work which are leading to the expression of inherited predisposition.

In Britain, figures for the prevalence of childhood obesity are both more modest and fairly consistent, ranging between 2 and 10 per cent depending on age, sex, and social class, and are quite similar to figures for European countries and the Antipodes. There is as yet no evidence of a dramatic increase of obesity among British children and adolescents. In all these countries, children from less-well-educated homes seem to have a greater prevalence of obesity. There does appear to be a problem of a different order in the United States when compared with other countries. However this leaves no room for complacency because the 'American' lifestyle and its consequences tends to spread elsewhere.

CAUSES OF OBESITY

Genetic

The evidence that genetic factors are important in determining the degree of adiposity comes from several sources. Family studies demonstrate that fat parents tend to have fat children, and that two fat parents are even more likely to have fat offspring. For a number of years, controversy has existed as to whether this is due to genetic factors or to the life-styles of the families. Studies comparing identical and fraternal twins have tended to produce conflicting answers, but the balance of opinion is coming round to the view that genetic factors play an important but not exclusive role in determining familial obesity.

Environmental

The evidence that environmental factors have a role in the causation of obesity is borne out by many studies which show that obesity is at least to some extent determined by life-style and eating habits. Sedentary populations on high calorie intakes have a greater incidence of obesity. In some communities, changing social patterns or emigration have resulted in dramatic changes in the degree of adiposity. Interesting sex differences and reversals of relative obesity at certain ages also indicate that there are very important environmental effects on the amount of fat accumulated.

The physical activity, or lack of it, in modern western children caused by changes in life-style may well be a contributing factor to the increases in childhood obesity. Obese children are probably less physically fit than lean children but it is not clear whether this is cause or effect.

The amount of television watching by children is said to be an important factor in the United States. American children spend on average as much time watching television as attending school. This may not be entirely due to reduced physical activity, since television watching is often associated with the intake of alarming quantities of junk-foods such as sugar-coated cereals, candy bars, cakes, and sugared beverages. The television programmes themselves are frequently interspersed with advertisements for these foods, which encourages further energy intake. Television watching seems to combine high energy intake with low energy expenditure. It is possible that the association is indirect; children who are fat may shun or be shunned by other children and may be forced into excessive television watching. It may be that, as with an increase in energy intake, a general decline in physical activity causes obesity in those children who are genetically predisposed to accumulate adipose tissue. There is probably a vicious cycle in which children who get fat because of a combination of inactivity and excessive food intake become even more inactive. Such children will thus be increasingly hypoactive, partly because of the stigma attached to their physical appearance and partly because they find mobility difficult.

Genetic–environmental interactions

It may be the case that whereas genetic/metabolic factors determine which children are most vulnerable to becoming fat, it is the general pattern of eating and exercise which determines how many individuals will actually become overweight. It is also possible that individuals with an extreme risk of obesity will get fat on quite low energy intakes. In others the amount eaten may be the crucial factor in determining whether they become fat. All clinicians will have had experience of patients who have been fat at some time in their lives but who subsequently lose their overweight. One would not expect this to happen if the degree of adiposity was entirely genetically and metabolically determined. It is quite probable that the more homogeneous lifestyles are within a society, the more genetic predisposition will dominate as the causative factor.

Psychological factors

While this is not the place to discuss the very complex neurological and psychological factors which determine eating behaviour, there are some aspects of this fascinating area which may be of interest to the general reader.

The basic mechanisms which underlie the process of eating are located in the hypothalamus of the brain, which contains centres both for hunger and satiety, responsive to a variety of stimuli (Fig. 8.2). In man, as opposed to animals, there are powerful cognitive factors which after infancy may override the more primitive visceral responses.

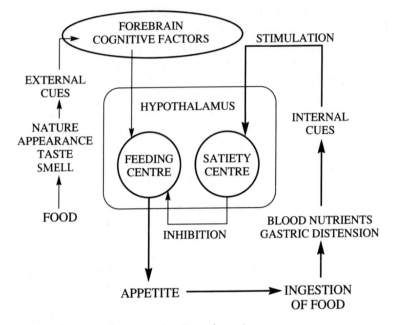

Fig. 8.2. Effects of various stimuli on the eating process.

It was thought for a time that obesity was due to overeating secondary to a mismatch or misinterpretation of so-called eating cues. External cues are stimuli such as the appearance, smell, or taste of food, whereas internal cues are the sensations normally interpreted as hunger or satiation. That such cues exist and play an important part in eating behaviour seems beyond dispute but it is no longer believed that their disturbance causes obesity. These ideas have become the basis for much behaviour-modification management.

One valuable concept, that of restrained and unrestrained eaters, has emerged. A restrained eater is an individual who consciously or unconsciously, as a result of conditioning, limits the amount of food ingested below complete satiation, whereas an unrestrained eater ingests to the point of complete satiation. Most individuals who become restrained eaters may have a fear or distaste for becoming obese. The extreme end of this spectrum may be anorexia nervosa.

Cognitive factors may therefore play an important part in determining the degree of adiposity of individuals, due to the strong social pressures against obesity in the general population.

Young children are by nature unrestrained eaters but peer pressures force at least some to control the amount they ingest. Parents who are themselves restrained eaters may ensure that their children do not eat to the point where they become obese. These factors may explain how some families with the genetic potential for obesity remain lean, whereas others succumb to their genes.

The dietary intake of an obese person may vary from low to high in different states of adiposity. Someone who has just lost weight from a diet may eat voraciously if unrestrained, until the body returns to its accustomed state of fatness. Some mechanism may then act on the internal cue system to reduce the amount ingested. An obese individual may be restraining food intake once obese so that no further increase in adiposity occurs but insufficiently to lose weight. In both situations the diet will be normal or even low in energy. Some lean people with high rates of metabolism may be unrestrained eaters but on the other hand some lean people are only lean by virtue of the fact that they are restraining their dietary intake.

CONSEQUENCES OF CHILDHOOD OBESITY

During childhood

There is a significant social stigma associated with being obese. Fat people are the victims of prejudice and discrimination. It is generally perceived that to be fat is somehow 'unhealthy' and that the fat person is in some way at fault. Approval of leanness has reached a point where obesity is regarded as evidence of 'degeneracy', with obese individuals becoming a despised, down-trodden, and even persecuted minority. Schoolchildren suffer the most and will admit that they are teased and tormented by peers and even by teachers. Yet diet is for some children an even less acceptable alternative. Most obese individuals are not emotionally disturbed, although adolescents may have a poor image of themselves and become depressed. This may be a result of futile attempts to slim.

Morbid obesity is fortunately quite rare in childhood. Most cases of very gross obesity in this age period are children with Prader-Willi syndrome or some other specific pathological entity. It is among this group of children that harmful or potentially life threatening complications, such as orthopaedic complications, skin conditions, the alveolar-hypoventilation syndrome (Pick-wickian syndrome), or cardiomyopathy (heart failure), can be expected to occur. These problems occur very rarely in children who are merely plump, and their prevalence should not be exaggerated.

Long-term effects

Although the statistical association between obesity and vascular disease seems to be beyond question, it is by no means certain that there is a direct causal relationship. When other risk factors such as hypertension and abnormal lipid patterns are excluded, obesity on its own does not appear to be very strongly associated with morbidity. On the other hand strong correlations exist with high LDL-cholesterol, low HDL-cholesterol, and hypertension, which are all undoubted risk factors for vascular disease.

SHOULD WE TREAT CHILDHOOD OBESITY?

What is to be done with children who are already fat? Young, fat children whose food intakes are determined by their parents can be made to lose weight by 'involuntary dieting', but anyone who has tried to cope with older, 'free-range' children will be aware of the difficulties involved in maintaining weight loss. In general unless a number of criteria are fulfilled it is an uphill struggle of doubtful value. The child should genuinely wish to become thinner and the parents should also be strongly motivated. If either parent is fat they should be willing to try to reduce their own obesity. In cases of familial obesity, unless there is a determination to change both eating and exercise patterns for the whole family, attempts at weight reduction in an individual child are largely a waste of time.

Which children should be dieted?

Given that most fat children placed on diets fail to maintain permanent weight loss there is a good case for a selective approach. Unless the parents of young children evince a genuine desire for their child to lose weight there is little to be gained from attempting to force the issue. Similarly unless older children themselves want to become slim there is little real chance of success. The trouble is that often both remaining fat and submitting to draconian diets are equally unacceptable. Little wonder that obesity has been labelled the 'miserable condition'.

In some situations, a more positive stance is indicated. Children with a family history of vascular disease or diabetes are particularly at risk, and it is legitimate to warn of the health hazards. Similarly children with a genuinely raised blood pressure or with a family history of hypertension should have firmer advice. Care needs to be taken in interpreting blood pressure readings in fat children because false, high readings are common.

Children presenting themselves for weight reduction are worth an effort but even here the proportion of failures remains high.

Dietary treatment

Treatment of childhood obesity using dietary manipulation would appear simple; however, in practice it can be extremely difficult. Children find it difficult to follow dietary regimes which set them apart from other children, and they need a great deal of support from their families. If overweight parents are unwilling to change their dietary habits, there will be little chance of the overweight child changing his/her eating pattern.

The success rates for treatment of childhood obesity are low. The ideal is to prevent obesity in the first place, and emphasis should be placed on healthy eating for the whole family, establishing good food habits in early childhood. This, however, does not solve the immediate problem of the overweight child, and dietary treatment must be considered.

Very-low-calorie, liquid diets (less than 600 kcal) are currently popular among the obese adult population and are advertised and marketed in every health-food shop and newspaper. They claim to promote rapid weight loss. We do not wish to discuss the pitfalls of these diets in relation to adults but must stress that the diets are not suitable for infants and children. There are many different very-low-calorie, liquid diets on the market today. None have been designed specifically for children. They are all low in energy, some are low in protein, and the balance of vitamins and minerals is unsuitable for the growing child. They can lead to nutritional deficiencies and poor growth. The liquid diet does not promote a long-term, healthy, eating pattern which is necessary for children to remain stable after weight loss.

Another category of very-low-calorie diets is based on 'normal' foods and aims to provide very low energy intakes, for example 300, 400, or 600 kcal daily. These are also unsuitable for children. The low energy intake makes it virtually impossible for the child to consume adequate protein, vitamins, and minerals, and long-term use will certainly impair a child's growth. It should be noted that these diets are very inflexible, unpalatable, and difficult to follow.

Other forms of dietary treatment include the many different 'fad diets' such as the 'F' plan, Scarsdale, egg, grapefruit, or Mars bar diets. They have transient notoriety with often exaggerated claims for their effectiveness. Some are, however, well-balanced and with slight modification can be suitable for children, but others are not acceptable. Before considering one of these diets for a child a careful assessment must be made to ensure that it provides a good nutritional balance. The overall energy should not be less than 1000 kcal, and care must be taken when giving high-fibre diets to young children, as discussed in Chapter 2.

A sensible, healthy, eating plan consisting of low-energy but high-nutrient dense foods is preferable to any of the above. Calorie counting is not usually necessary, although it can be a good way of achieving a balanced diet. Most dietitians would recommend that a child follows a nutritionally balanced diet, avoiding excess. The recommendations for a healthy, weight-reducing diet for children include the avoidance of fried foods, high-energy, low-nutrient dense snack foods, and concentrated sugary foods. The children should be encouraged to eat only at meal-times and recognized snack times. Puddings should be substituted by fresh fruit or other low-calorie desserts, and high-sugar squash and fizzy drinks should be replaced by their low-calorie counterparts. An example of a suitable diet for children wishing to lose weight is shown in Table 8.1 and the accompanying menu plan (Table 8.2). This is the type of diet used by the authors and forms a basis for dietary education. The families will require further information regarding suitable cereal

Table 8.1. Weight-reducing diet suitable for children

Stop Foods high in calories to be avoided	Steady Foods quite high in calories but necessary for growth	Go Food low in calories and can be eaten freely

All fatty and fried foods
Butter, margarine, lard, dripping, oils.[1]
Crisps
Chips
Fried vegetables
Cream
Condensed milk
Evaporated milk
All sugary foods
  sugar
  jam, marmalade
  honey, syrup
  sweets, chocolates
  toffee
  ice cream
  cakes, biscuits
  puddings,
  pies and pastries
  sweetened drinks
	Protein foods
	Lean meat, fish
	Eggs
	Cheese
	Baked beans
	Beans, pulses, nuts
	Milk, skimmed or semi[2]
	Bread and cereals[2]
		Vegetables—all
		  raw
		  boiled
		  steamed
		Salads
		Fruit
		  fresh
		  frozen
		Squash/drinks
		  low-calorie
		  tea
		  coffee
		Sweeteners
		  low-calorie
		
		Herbs, spices
		Seasonings

[1] Other than in allowances.
[2] Within allowances.

Table 8.2. Menu plan based on a diet in Table 8.1

Breakfast	Small glass of unsweetened fruit-juice Wholegrain cereal, milk from allowance and/or wholemeal toast with margarine Tea or coffee, milk from allowance, no sugar
Mid-morning snack	Fresh fruit (if wanted) Low calorie squash
Lunch	Lean meat or fish Vegetables or salad Fresh fruit or low-calorie yogurt Low-calorie squash or water
Mid-afternoon snack	Cup of tea or low-calorie squash or fizzy drink Wholemeal toast with margarine or fresh fruit
Evening meal	Lean meat or cheese or egg Vegetables or salad 1 small portion of boiled potato Fresh fruit or unsweetened canned fruit Low calorie squash or drink of milk from daily allowance
Bed-time snack	Tea or low calorie squash Wholemeal toast or wholegrain cereal if allowances permit

exchanges, low-calorie recipes, snack and packed-lunch ideas. If the child usually has a school lunch the school will need to be contacted and a suitable meal requested.

If a strict regime is necessary and the child's food intake falls below 1000 calories, vitamin and possibly mineral supplements should be given. All children on dietary restriction should be monitored carefully to ensure that their overall nutrition and growth is not impaired. Some drastic weight-losing programmes may lead to a fall in linear growth. Very often there is a dramatic initial loss of weight with dieting. Unfortunately this is mainly due to loss of lean body mass. The resulting fall in metabolic rate may make further weight loss more difficult.

Exercise is an important factor in helping a child to lose weight. They should be encouraged to participate in the usual school sports and games as well as to take up some other forms of exercise out of school. Some obese children are reluctant to take part in sport because of their body habitus. In some cases it may help to start weight reduction and to implement an exercise programme after a few weeks when a better shape has been attained. Exercise should be graduated and this may begin with walking instead of travelling by bus or car. Other good forms of exercise include swimming, jogging and gymnastics. It is important that exercise is taken at least three times a week and that it continues for a sufficiently long period. Short bursts of exercise are anaerobic and do not burn fat. Aerobic exercise will burn fat and increase metabolic rate during exercise and possibly for some time afterwards. Exercise will not only assist weight loss but will also promote a feeling of well-being.

Children following a weight-reducing programme usually need a great deal of support, and regular follow-up can be an important factor in their success. Follow-up should preferably not take place in a hospital clinic setting. It may be more appropriate in school or the local health clinic because obesity should not be stigmatized as a disease but as a correctable state. Group sessions can help some children but not all.

Rapid weight loss is not necessary and may be harmful. A slow, gradual loss is preferable or the maintenance of a stable weight which falls relatively as the child gains height. The occasional older child may actually continue to lose weight after an ideal weight is reached and may develop a state similar to mild anorexia nervosa.

The overweight infant should be dealt with in a completely different way, and strict dietary regimes are not appropriate for the child under the age of 1 year and probably not before 2 years of age. Simple modifications should be made to the feeding pattern, and there should be some alterations in the types of foods offered, the emphasis being on a gradual introduction of a healthy diet as outlined in the weaning section of Chapter 1. Suggestions for modifying the feeds of the overweight baby, weanling, and toddler include:

1. Infant formulas should be correctly prepared and not over-concentrated.
2. Avoid over-frequent and excessive feeding.
3. Devise a feeding plan giving times and volumes of feed.

4. A small-hole teat can be useful in slowing down the rate of ingestion.

5. Water should be offered when the baby is thirsty, not more milk feeds.

6. Solids must not be added to bottle feeds.

7. Sugar should not be added to solid foods.

8. Low-energy dense solids with a high nutrient content should be given in preference to high-energy dense solids. Examples of these include pureed fruit, vegetables, wholegrain cereals and lean meats.

Behaviour modification

Attempts to alter the eating patterns of children has led to the development of behaviourally based strategies which have had varying success. Unfortunately the field has become somewhat jargon-laden and it is now very difficult to write about it without using jargon. There are a variety of systems but most include:

1. Positive reinforcement and negative reinforcement. This means, in effect, use of both rewards and punishment.

2. So-called contingency management which ensures that participants understand the material presented to them.

3. A record is kept by parents and children of weight, food intake, and their reactions to meals.

4. The provision of ideal eating models for the rest of the family.

5. Agreeing a contract in which parents deposit a sum of money with the therapists which is returned in tranches as goals are achieved.

6. Incentive systems, whereby the child may actually be rewarded for reaching goals.

Acquiring self-management skills using cognitive-behaviour-modification methods are relatively more successful in older children, whereas parental management is more important in the younger ones. Behaviour-modification programmes have been used in the school setting, within obesity clinics, and as a component of family-based programmes.

Family-based treatment

Family-based systems are based on observations that children lost similar amounts of weight during the initial phases of weight-reducing schedules but those with whom the parents had been involved showed a more sustained response.

There are three essential components to the treatment programme:

1. Diet using the 'traffic light' system. Food is divided into 11 categories and further subdivided into green (food with less than 20 calories per average serving), yellow (amber-food with about 20 calories per average serving), and red (food exceeding the caloric density of the 'yellow' foods), the colours corresponding to 'Go', 'Cautious' and 'Stop' with obvious implications. Four servings of 'red' foods are allowed per week. The child is expected to keep a written record of the various foods ingested in their appropriate categories. Parents are expected to praise children for keeping to the restrictions on the various categories of foods.

2. An exercise programme.

3. Behavioural treatment programme for parents and older children.

A comprehensive programme of this nature requires special skills and is likely to be costly. Since the long-term outlook for familial obesity is at present so poor the approach certainly deserves careful consideration.

PREVENTING CHILDHOOD OBESITY

No one can doubt that it is a disadvantage to be overweight whether or not it is a significant risk factor for subsequent vascular disease. There seems to be a strong case for discouraging young children from becoming overweight if this can be achieved. Those who believe that obesity is largely genetically determined may take the view that this is not possible. We prefer the view that in at least some children, the overall adiposity of the population can be prevented from rising by sensible policies, even if some individuals very strongly predisposed to obesity will get fat irrespective of environmental factors. The experience of the United States where there appears to be an explosion of obesity among both children and adults is something we ought to try to prevent.

Although for a time it was thought that infantile obesity might programme individuals to a lifetime of overweight, it has become clear that, except in some special instances, events during the first months of life probably have little bearing on later body habitus, provided that the infant is fed either breast milk or correctly prepared infant formula and is not commenced on high calorie solids too early. Most very plump infants slim down during early childhood and true infantile obesity persisting into adulthood is very rare. Apart from following the laid down principles for infant feeding, there seems little justification for the introduction of policies aimed at preventing overweight in babies.

Much more important seems to be the post-toddler period. The age period from 2 years to 6 years is the leanest time of life, so the onset of obesity during this time is an important matter which may have a permanent effect. Significant obesity begins to appear in the preschoolchild. Just why some children not previously fat begin to put on weight is not really understood. Metabolically based theories do not explain this since one would expect individuals predetermined to be fat to be so from the start. It seems prudent to assume that the pattern of eating and activity has something to do with it.

This is the period during which children may adopt particular patterns of eating and physical activity. Parents who find it convenient to place a child in front of a television or video screen with a bag of crisps and a bottle of pop should be aware that this is an unsound practice with possible long-term, harmful consequences. Social policy which leads to the trapping of families into this sort of life-style needs to be re-examined.

Parents should be encouraged to avoid excessive high calorie and fat intakes in their children's diets and to discourage snacking on 'empty calorie' foods and drinks. The promotion of a life-style for the whole family which involves a reasonable amount of physical activity is to be encouraged. Particularly if parents are overweight, they should be encouraged to re-examine their own eating and activity patterns.

The prevalence of obesity increases sharply after adolescence and goes on increasing into adult life. Paradoxically some fat children may slim down during adolescence, presumably because of cognitive pressures. Many simply decide that they will not be fat any longer. A population of 'restrained eaters' emerges, people who consciously or unconsciously restrain their intake of energy to achieve a desirable body habitus but who would, presumably because of the nature of their genetically determined metabolism, become obese otherwise. This subset of the popultion at least demonstrates that some individuals can alter their body habitus by dietary means.

9

The schoolchild and adolescent

SCHOOLCHILDREN and adolescents in Britain are taller and heavier than in the past and the secular trend for increasing body size continues. This has been interpreted as evidence that the population is healthier than ever before and that nutritional standards are good and improving. However there is growing concern that recent changes in social policy and in life-style may put at least some schoolchildren and adolescents at risk because they could have subclinical nutritional deficiencies. On the other hand there is concern that the increased intake of energy and fat, particularly animal fat, may be predisposing the younger generation to an increased risk of vascular disease.

THE SCHOOLCHILD

Many changes occur in a child's life when formal education begins. The noon meal is frequently taken at school, and the environment in which food is eaten will be very different from home. Getting to school on time can interfere with breakfast, children may be unwilling get up in time to eat, and some parents may not provide their children with an adequate breakfast.

Schoolchildren have changing nutritional needs which vary according to the level of growth, and various nutritional problems can arise. These include undernutrition, which is characterized by poor growth and anaemia, particularly in children from low income families or where a poor diet is eaten. Rickets is seen in Asian children and children who are on odd diets.

Children who have had iron-deficiency anaemia should be encouraged to eat foods rich in iron, folate, and vitamin C.

Unfortunately these are often unpopular with children and many refuse to eat red meats, green vegetables, or fresh fruits. Alternative foods or methods of serving high iron foods can be found.

SCHOOL MEALS

In the 1980 Education Act there were major changes made to the laws governing the provision of school meals. Local authorities are no longer required to provide meals of a certain nutritional standard at a fixed price. Prior to 1980 the school meal was required to provide a third of a child's nutritional intake. The consequences of these changes are:

1. There is no guarantee that meals provided meet a required nutritional standard, and therefore that the child will receive an adequate meal.

2. Wide choice designed to attract custom will not educate children into healthy eating habits and in many cases food choices are high in fat and sugar and low in fibre and vitamins.

3. Children are free to spend dinner money elsewhere.

On the positive side many schools are working hard to offer healthy meals that are still attractive to children, and many are adopting local healthy-eating policies. Some school-meal departments are linking with teachers in an attempt to provide nutrition education.

Problems with school meals include inadequate time available, particularly for young children who are slow eaters. If a child has to queue for a long time to obtain his meal there may be little time left to eat it and the choice of food may be limited. In many schools there is a lack of suitable meals for minority groups including vegetarians. In older schoolchildren the temptation to skip school lunch and eat out at a fast food take-away can mean that an unbalanced meal is eaten, and parents may be unaware of what their children are eating and are therefore not able to make up deficiencies at home. All these problems are compounded by the growing tendency for convenience foods to be eaten in homes. Particularly at risk are children from less privileged homes. While official pronouncements based on surveys have been reassuring, this is a situation that requires continuous monitoring, and until a clearer picture emerges of what schoolchildren actually eat, anxiety must remain.

THE ADOLESCENT

Nutritional needs

Because of the rapid growth spurt during adolescence, energy and nutrient requirements are greatly increased. The peak period of growth is between 11 and 14 years of age for girls and between 13 and 16 years of age for boys. Girls accumulate relatively more fat body mass, and boys more lean body mass. Overall, boys increase their total body mass much more dramatically than girls and so RDA values deviate increasingly from about 10 years of age. The amount of energy required will depend on the degree of physical activity in which the individual is engaged, and this varies considerably. Specific nutrients which could become deficient include calcium, iron, and zinc.

Delayed puberty

A number of children who have previously been growing normally will show a deceleration in their height velocity just before the normal onset of puberty. This will often be associated with delay in the development of secondary sexual characteristics. This condition is usually referred to as delayed pubertal growth spurt.

Some variation in height centiles may occur as the child nears puberty, because a probably genetically determined biological variable—the age of onset of puberty—makes itself felt. Thus children with delayed puberty who are otherwise normal may show a fall in the position of the centile chart which will later be made good as the child catches up. Such children are destined to be shorter than their peers from about 10 to 18 years of age. Boys take longer to catch up than girls.

Although most children with delayed puberty are normal, children with nutritional problems who are growing slowly often have delay in puberty. Children with a range of chronic illnesses are much more likely to manifest this phenomenon.

Nutritional supplementation may have some effect in promoting the growth spurt and is worth trying. It is important to assess the child's current nutritional intake and to identify areas of nutritional deficiency or low nutrient intake. The problem is sometimes simply an energy deficiency with the child taking adequate quantities of other nutrients. If this is the problem, advice should be given on increasing the energy content of the diet using high-calorie foods such as fats and sugars. This needs to be worked out carefully with the child and parents and 'normal' foods should

Table 9.1. Some dietary supplements

Carbohydrate	Fat	Protein
Sugar	Butter	Skimmed-milk powder
Glucose	Margarine	Casilan (Farleys)
Polycal (Cow & Gate)	Cream	Maxipro HBV (SHS[1])
Polycose (Abbott)	Calogen (SHS[1])	Protifar (Cow & Gate)
Caloreen (Roussel)	Liquigen (SHS[1])	ProMod (Abbott)
Hycal (Beechams)		Forceval (Unigreg)
Fortical (Cow & Gate)	**Carbohydrate + Fat**	
Maxijul (SHS[1])	Duocal (SHS[1])	
Nutritionally Complex Drinks		
Whole milk	**Desserts**	
Homemade milkshakes	Maxisorb (SHS[1])	
e.g. using milk,	Formance (Abbott)	
yoghurt, ice cream, fruit	Protipudding (Cow & Gate)	
	Soups	
Complan (Farleys)	Maxisorb (SHS[1])	
Carnation Build-Up (Nestle)	Complan-Chicken (Farleys)	
Fortimel (Cow & Gate)	Carnation Build-Up	
Fortisip (Cow & Gate)	Chicken, Mushroom	
Nutrifruit (Wyeth)	(Nestle)	
Supplement (Wyeth)		
Fresubin (Fresenius)		
Ensure (Abbott)		

[1] Scientific Hospital Supplies.
Many dietary supplements are not suitable for children unless modified and should only be used under dietetic supervision.

be used as a first choice. If further calorie supplements are required there are a variety of special products available (see Table 9.1) in the form of glucose polymers and fat emulsions which may be used with care and can be incorporated into the child's diet disguised in milk drinks, fruit juices, or other foods.

In those children where the overall nutritional intake is low, similar advice should be given. More 'complete food' should be used as supplements. Adding milk powder or milk to a wide variety of foods and drinks is often a cheap and effective supplement. Specialized complete food supplements (Table 9.1), in the form of 'milk-shakes', desserts, and soups are available and are usually well liked by children. These supplements often require modification and should only be used under dietetic supervision. Some are prescribable, others are available directly from the manufacturer, and some are easily purchased from a pharmacy or supermarket. Vitamin and mineral supplements may also be necessary.

It is important to use these supplements in conjunction with the child's usual diet and to encourage an increase in normal foods as far as possible. Regular follow-up is important to check height and weight and to assess the overall nutritional content of the diet. It has been our practice to arrange dietetic follow-up until supplements are no longer required.

Adolescent eating patterns

Adolescence is a time in which a transition occurs from child to adult eating behaviour. Experimentation with new eating habits is common before settling down. Some adolescents may opt for vegetarianism out of serious principle and they should be given every assistance in establishing their new way of life on a sound nutritional footing.

Food faddism based on misconceptions about food may lead to poor food choice and sub-optimal nutrition. Fortunately most fads are short-term and have no lasting ill effects. Nutrition education is important because of its role in preventing adult disease and because it provides a sound basis for future parenthood. However, due to the nature of adolescence this is difficult, as anything suggested by an adult is likely to be viewed with suspicion and ignored at least at first.

Excessive anxiety about obesity may lead to distorted eating and exercise patterns. Bulimia and anorexia nervosa are among the disorders which may result. These are basically psychiatric conditions. The currently favored method for treating anorexia is still a matter of controversy because of its strongly coercive element, but diet plays only a peripheral role.

Anorexia nervosa

This term describes a state in which aversion to food is global and so severe as to cause dangerous weight loss. Anorexia nervosa is associated with amenorrhoea in girls, in whom the condition is more common. Some cases of prepubertal anorexia nervosa occur.

If there is a threat to life because of malnutrition, admission to hospital is necessary, and the dietary management in conjunction with psychiatric treatment comprises achieving a safe weight by providing adequate nutrition. The regime may include nasogastric feeding, dietary supplements, and a graded reintroduction of food through meals, with a progressive increase in their nutritional content.

DIET AND BEHAVIOUR

There are considerable attractions both for parents and health professionals in trying to ascribe often intractable and worrying problems to causes which might be amenable to relatively simple solutions. Parents with children who are not achieving what might be expected of them, or those whose behaviour has become intolerable, are likely to grasp at the straws provided by potential 'cures' which are simple, cheap, and apparently harmless. It is not easy for parents to accept that under-achievement or disturbed behaviour might be inherited or the result of unsatisfactory rearing methods.

Establishing a scientifically valid link between dietary deficiencies (or excess) and conditions which are usually multifactorial in their origins is a notoriously tricky area for investigation.

We have already noted that food intolerance has on scanty evidence been held responsible for behaviour problems in children, and dietary additives are incriminated, with little justification, in so-called hyperactivity. Other dietary factors which are thought to have effects on behaviour and intelligence in schoolchildren are sucrose and supposed vitamin deficiency.

Sucrose intake and behaviour

In recent years there have been a number of anecdotal reports implicating dietary sugars as a factor in behaviour problems in children. In particular, sucrose has been singled out as the main culprit. The basis for this hypothesis is the claim that meals high in sucrose stimulate excessive production of insulin with a consequent dip of blood glucose to symptomatic levels resulting in impaired behaviour.

It has been claimed that foods rich in sugar can cause antisocial behaviour and delinquency. The data on which these claims are based are open to many criticisms, and certainly provide no proper basis for formulating policy. If anything they seem to demonstrate aberrant eating patterns in delinquents rather than a causative relationship. This sort of claim is very difficult to either prove or disprove but a recent review of the subject has concluded that there is no substantive evidence to support it.

The supposed effects of sugary foods on hyperactivity are twofold. In the first instance it is claimed that sucrose may actually cause hyperkinesis. On the other hand, there have been claims that sucrose may aggravate symptoms in already hyperactive children. There have been a number of reports of postprandial symptoms suggestive of hypoglycaemia. Much of this is as a result of self-diagnosis or diagnosis by individuals who do not have appropriate clinical skills, and the terms pseudohypoglycaemia or non hypoglycaemia have been coined to describe it.

It is claimed that not only does sucrose ingestion produce the symptoms normally associated with hypoglycaemia (i.e. sweating, palpitations, piloerection, and trembling) but also a whole

range of less specific behavioural symptoms such as mood
change, depression, poor cerebration, and even delinquent
behaviour. There is little or no valid evidence to support the
views that high sucrose intake is an important cause of behaviour
disturbance either by causing hypoglycaemia or through some
other mechanism.

VITAMIN AND MINERAL INTAKE OF SCHOOLCHILDREN

It is generally believed that the diets commonly eaten by children
in this country provide an adequate intake of vitamins and
minerals. Surveys of the diets of schoolchildren have not revealed
significant deficits and there has been more concern in recent
years because of the possibility of excess nutrient intake particularly of energy and saturated fats.

There remains a school of thought that all is not well with the
diets of children, quite apart from the risk factors for obesity
and vascular disease already discussed. The abandonment of the
principle of free meals at school, the provision of 'freedom of
choice' for youngsters regarding the meals they buy, and the
growth of the junk-food industry worry many people, but so far
no real evidence has been produced that any harm results in the
short or medium term. There have been recent studies suggesting that the diets of at least some children are deficient and that
supplementing them with vitamins and minerals may improve
non-verbal intelligence. These findings are at best tentative and
it will need much more evidence to prove them valid.

Subclinical deficiencies of vitamins are regularly incriminated
as possible causes of disease and dysfunction. Linus Pauling
believed that ascorbic acids in large doses could prevent the
common cold. It has been suggested that inadequate vitamin
intake during pregnancy might be a factor in the pathogenesis of
spina bifida. 'Mega-vitamin' treatment for all sorts of ills are
fashions which come and go.

Uncontrolled vitamin intake is not without risk. Fat-soluble
vitamins in particular can be dangerous. Excess intake of vitamin A can cause hypertension and brain injury, whereas vitamin

D poisoning will lead to hypercalcaemia and renal damage. Water-soluble vitamins are safer than fat-soluble vitamins because any excess intake is excreted in the urine. Huge doses of ascorbic acid can cause haematuria, and a massive intake of pyridoxine has been associated with peripheral neuropathy.

Preparations of vitamins can be freely bought from health food shops and pharmacies. Provided parents do not overdose their children with Vitamins A or D it is unlikely that this form of supplementation will do much harm. There seems at present no justification for providing multiple vitamin/mineral supplementation at public expense.

10

Special diets

SPECIAL diets play an important role in the management of a number of diseases. They need careful planning, have to be tailored to the individual needs of the patient, and long-term clinical and biochemical monitoring is necessary to ensure adequate nutrition. We are not aiming to give a comprehensive account of this field, but we believe that health workers who come in contact with children on such diets, and parents who have children on treatment should have some basic knowledge of the principles which underlie their management. The diets are complicated and should be carried out by a specialist team which should include a paediatrician, paediatric dietitian, and where appropriate, a biochemist with special expertise in the field. In some conditions other health workers should be part of the team e.g. physiotherapists in cystic fibrosis. Ideally outpatient consultations should be carried out jointly by the members of the team.

Regular, careful measurement and assessment of physical and intellectual development is a cornerstone of succesful management. The most important evidence that the diet is satisfactory is the growth of the child. Units providing for the care of these children must have the ability to carry out body measurements (anthropometric studies) with precision.

The emotional needs of families (including siblings) with children on special and complicated diets may be considerable, requiring much community support by specially trained personnel. Wherever possible a health visitor or similarly trained person should be attached to the laboratory and/or clinic, seeing the family with the paediatrician and acting as a liaison between the central service and the community. Such a person can be of enormous benefit in the guidance of health professionals and education service regarding the needs of the child. By regular visits to the homes, far better control of diet is possible, misunderstandings can be resolved, and by providing a link between families and various parts of the service, an esprit de corps may be created not otherwise easy to achieve. The brothers and sisters of children on diets may actually feel neglected and their needs should be actively considered. If possible they should be made to feel part of the team.

A hospital-based social worker who attends the special clinic can acquire a very useful understanding of the problems of these often stressed families and may be of great assistance in easing their difficulties. Ideally dietitians should be ready to make home visits regularly. Unfortunately constraints on resources do not always allow for this. Nevertheless the occasional visit can be enormously beneficial.

All this expertise and experience can only be attained if there is a reasonable concentration of patients. In some rare disorders, cases may be scattered over a wide area. It is highly desirable for many reasons that all such children should be seen from time to time at the specialist centre. Management of some conditions is evolving all the time. There are constant changes in what is regarded as 'best practice' which pass along the grape-vine and will not be known to most doctors and dietitians. New products which make diets easier to cope with are 'arriving' regularly. Parents with children on unusual diets being treated away from specialist centres often complain that they are not kept abreast of such developments.

Dealing with many cases gives the specialist paediatricians and dietitians a 'feel' they do not otherwise possess. The furtherance of knowledge, which most parents would wish to see, also requires some concentration of cases.

Unfortunately there is sometimes a reluctance to part with what are regarded as 'interesting cases'. A team approach to management is the essence of success. This is emphatically not an area for the 'rugged individualist', consultant paediatrician giving orders to others. We have seen many examples of children receiving less than optimal care because of this. Some form of 'shared care' system may be evolved between the local paediatrician and dietetic service and the specialist unit. Parents of children with rare diseases have a right to demand that they be referred to specialist centres.

INBORN ERRORS OF METABOLISM

Of those inborn errors of metabolism which are amenable to treatment, dietary management is crucial to almost all. In many cases this involves eliminating or reducing from the diet some component of normal nutrition which cannot be properly metabolized (e.g. phenylalanine in phenylketonuria). In others, it is a matter of supplementing the diet with a nutrient that may be deficient as a consequence of the enzyme defect (e.g. glucose in acyl-CoA-dehydrogenase defects). A third and particularly interesting group of disorders are those in which the requirements for certain vitamins or enzyme co-factors are greatly increased and huge doses of normal vitamins may be needed (e.g. biotin in biotinidase deficiency). This last group is particularly rewarding because effective treatment with a dietary agent is so simple and effective (see Fig. 10.1). In a fourth group of inborn disorders, diet plays a very important but subsidiary role in management (e.g. cystic fibrosis).

The increasing number of treatable diseases and increasing complexity of management combined with their rarity is making it mandatory for such children to be seen in a centre which specializes in metabolic disorders. Optimal management may be difficult to achieve. The very ability to recognize that control is sub-optimal requires the skill that comes only from extensive experience.

Prevalence

Individually, treatable, inborn errors of metabolism are not common, but taken as a group they constitute a significant number of children with potential handicap, morbidity, and mortality who are entitled to expect optimal treatment in a

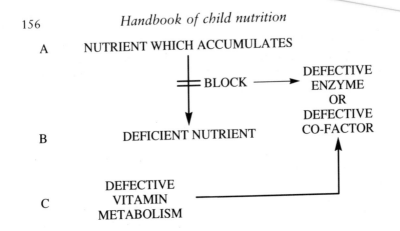

Fig. 10.1. Inborn errors of metabolism. Methods of treatment are: A, restrict nutrient, i.e. phenylalanine in phenylketonuria; B, provide extra nutrient, i.e. tyrosine in phenylketonuria; C, give large doses of vitamin, i.e. biotin in biotinidase activity.

wealthy country such as Britain. For each million people in the population there will be born each year about 30 children with a genetic disorder likely to benefit from dietary help (Table 10.1). With passage of time more conditions at present untreatable may become at least in part amenable to dietary management.

Hyperlipidaemia

Lipids (fats) may exist either as neutral fats which contain fatty acids and glycerol, or as cholesterol fats (esters).

The two main types of primary hyperlipidaemia encountered in childhood are Type 2A familial hypercholesterolaemia in which the cholesterol esters are increased in the blood, and Type 1 or familial lipoprotein lipase deficiency in which there is an increase in neutral fats which are present in the blood as droplets, chylomicrons. Chylomicrons may separate from a blood sample to form a creamy layer. Type 2A hyperlipidaemia is by far the most common inherited metabolic disorder, with an

Table 10.1. Frequency of genetic disorders amenable to dietary treatment (per million population)

Disease	Incidence (cases per annum)	Likely prevalence (children under 15 years)
Hyperlipidaemia type 2A	20	300
Cystic fibrosis	4	<60
Phenylketonuria	1	15
Other inborn errors	1	15
Totals	26	390

incidence of 1:500 in the population. Type 1 hyperlipidaemia is a much rarer condition.

Type 2A hyperlipidaemia (hypercholesterolaemia)

Type 2A hypercholesterolaemia is an autosomal dominant inherited disorder. Serum beta lipoproteins are found in increased amounts in the serum due to the defective removal of cholesterol. Most significantly, LDL-cholesterol is elevated from a very early age. As a consequence, the condition is associated with a high incidence of premature ischaemic heart disease. Early diagnosis and treatment can prevent this.

Children at risk are those from families where there is a history of someone having a heart attack at an early age or someone with a known raised serum cholesterol. Not all hypercholesterolaemia is due to this inherited defect. Most adults with raised LDL-cholesterol do not have type 2A hyperlipaemia. Nevertheless all children who have a parent or grandparent, aunt or uncle who developed early vascular disease should be screened for hyperlipaemia. If their serum cholesterol is raised they should follow a diet with reduced overall fat content and a high ratio of polyunsaturated to saturated fat.

As we have seen, in relation to healthy eating in general, monounsaturated fatty acids are gaining prominence because they promote the formation of HDL-cholesterol, and it may be that here too achieving a balance between polyunsaturated, monounsaturated, and saturated fatty acids will become important.

To compensate for the reduction in fat an increased carbohydrate intake is necessary, and complex carbohydrate foods such as wholegrain cereals, wholemeal bread, potato, pulses, fruit, and vegetables are preferable to concentrated, sugary carbohydrate foods. Soluble fibre found in high concentrations in oats and some beans have a cholesterol-lowering effect, more so than the predominantly insoluble fibre found in wheat bran.

Experience so far suggests that many children, particularly adolescents, do not follow their diets, and drug treatment with cholestyramine and other cholesterol-lowering preparations may be needed. Much depends on motivation and it is likely that a positive approach, with the setting up of well-staffed lipid clinics which start children on diets from an early age, will improve management. This is an area where parents groups could be very helpful.

It is important that the diet is followed for life and that the serum cholesterol levels are checked regularly as a way of monitoring dietary compliance. It is often difficult for a child to follow such a diet if the rest of the family eat differently. Dietary advice should be aimed at the whole family since the diet, which follows the COMA recommendations, will certainly do those not affected no harm.

It is surprising that a condition so common and potentially dangerous, yet treatable, has attracted little attention and that few resources are devoted to its management.

Because individuals with type 2A hypercholesterolaemia survive well into adult life it is possible for them to have children. In 1 in 250 000 families both parent will carry the abnormal gene. Half their children will thus inherit two abnormal genes for the condition and be homozygous. This is a devastating state which responds poorly to diet and leads to very severe vascular disease at an early age. Treatment includes plasmapheresis and small gut bypasses. Fortunately it is extremely rare, about two cases per million births.

Type 1 hyperlipidaemia

Type 1 lipoprotein lipase deficiency is an extremely rare auto-somal recessive disorder and appears to be particularly prevalent among consanguineous Asian couples. The basic defect is a deficiency in the aprotein C, which results in the inactivation of lipoprotein lipase and failure to clear chylomicrons at a normal rate. In infants and young children the clinical presentation includes failure to thrive, attacks of abdominal pain, eruptive xanthoma (skin lesions), and hepatosplenomegaly. The serum is milky in the fasting state with a gross elevation of triglyceride. The treatment is a very-low-fat diet with increased carbohydrate to ensure adequate energy intake. Medium chain triglycerides (MCT) can also be used to increase energy and more importantly to make the diet more palatable. Medium chain triglycerides are usually used as an oil for frying or coating foods. When absorbed, MTC does not form chylomicrons. As with all severely fat-restricted diets the child's intake of fat-soluble vitamins will be low and a vitamin supplement is necessary.

Cystic fibrosis

Cystic fibrosis is the commonest major autosomal recessive disorder found in Caucasian populations in the western world. The incidence in Britain ranges between 1:1600 and 1:2300 births. It affects males and females equally. It is a multi-organ disorder characterized by chronic pulmonary disease, pancreatic insufficiency, liver dysfunction, and abnormally high sweat electrolytes. The basic defect is still unknown but the manifesta-tions of the disease can be accounted for by a generalized dis-order of the exocrine and mucus-secreting glands. The clinical and pathological features are a direct consequence of obstruction of the small ducts by mucus.

Approximately 10 per cent of children with cystic fibrosis have meconium ileus at birth. The remainder are identified in early childhood with recurrent chest infections, failure to thrive, abdominal pain, and malabsorption. The diagnosis is confirmed by a raised concentration of sodium and chloride in the sweat on at least two tests. The radioimmune trypsin test is valid during the first weeks of life and has become the basis of a screening test for the condition.

The main problem in cystic fibrosis is respiratory. Severe chronic lung infection leads to a gradual deterioration in pulmonary function in most children. It is thought that maintaining good nutrition may delay the deterioration of lung function.

Nutritional problems are commonly due to the malabsorption related to the insufficiency of pancreatic enzymes, but poor appetite, inadequate food intake, and increased requirements due to recurrent infection also play their part. Some children with cystic fibrosis are said to have voracious appetites but this is usually not enough to compensate for the malabsorption.

The problems of malabsorption can be largely overcome by the use of pancreatic enzyme supplements, and the more modern preparations, Pancrease and Creon, are extremely effective. Dietary fat restriction is not usually necessary as long as adequate pancreatic enzyme supplements are given. The enzymes need to be taken with all food. Larger amounts are necessary with meals and less with snacks.

A normal to high fat intake should be encouraged since this will increase the energy content of the diet. High-energy snacks between meals, and dietary supplements in the form of milkshakes or glucose polymers are often necessary. There is also an increased requirement for protein, and high-protein foods should be encouraged. Fat-soluble vitamins and occasionally mineral and trace minerals may be given as supplements.

Because of the growing complexity of management and the problematic nature of some current therapy, children may require repeated stays in hospital. The treatment, including the administration of antibiotics, enzyme preparations, dietary supplements, and physiotherapy, takes up a great deal of time. The families need much help and support. The Cystic Fibrosis Research Trust offers support and advice.

Phenylketonuria

Phenylketonuria is an autosomal recessive disorder with an incidence of between 1:8000 to 1:10 000 births in Britain. It results from a deficiency of the enzyme phenylalanine hydroxylase, leading to failure of conversion of the essential amino acid phenylalanine to tyrosine. Consequently, there is an accumulation of phenylalanine in the blood, which if prolonged and sufficiently increased leads to brain damage. Treatment with a low phenylalanine diet prevents this. There appear to be different mutations (alleles) for phenylketonuria and not all cases are equally severe. Those requiring drastic protein restriction are said to have the 'classical' form of the disease whereas others are described as 'atypical' or to have hyperphenylalaninaemia. It has become apparent over the years that the range of protein restriction needed is wide and varies considerably from child to child.

In Britain all babies are screened for phenylketonuria between the sixth and tenth day of life. The blood test, commonly known as the 'Guthrie' test, is performed by the midwife, usually in the babies home. It is important that the test is done on or around the 6th day and not when the baby is born. The blood phenylalanine level will only be raised after feeding has been established and the baby has consumed some phenylalanine present in milk protein.

A blood phenylalanine level greater than 800 μmol/l is indicative of classical phenylketonuria. Normal blood levels may reach as high as 200 μmol/l. A blood level lower than 800 μmol/l but above the normal range indicates that the child has an atypical form of phenylketonuria. It sometimes happens, particularly in breast-fed babies, that blood levels are initially quite low, but on transfer to diets higher in phenylalanine, e.g. infant formula, serum levels rise to the point where dietary restriction is indicated. For this reason, all children with blood phenylalanine levels above the normal range should be referred to a specialist centre for further evaluation. Those with classical phenylketonuria will be treated immediately, while the borderline cases will be carefully followed.

A rare variant of phenylketonuria occurs, in which although the blood phenylalanine level responds to diet, brain damage continues. This is because the defect is of the co-factor, biopterin, which is necessary for important metabolic processes in the brain other than the conversion of phenylalanine to tyrosine. This condition does not respond to diet. All babies with high phenylalanine levels are automatically screened for the biopterin defect.

Treatment of phenylketonuria consists of a diet low in the amino acid phenylalanine. Phenylalanine is present is all proteins and these must therefore be removed from the diet. Certain amino acids in protein are essential and must therefore be replaced by a synthetic mixture of amino acids which does not include phenylalanine. Tyrosine, which is not normally an essential amino acid as it is normally synthesized from phenylalanine, becomes essential in individuals with phenylketonuria (see Fig. 10.1). It is therefore included in the amino-acid supplement. The diet must be balanced in every other respect and must contain adequate energy, vitamins, and minerals for growth.

In the baby this is achieved by using a specially prepared infant formula such as Minafen (Cow & Gate), Lofenalac (Mead Johnson), or Analog XP (Scientific Hospital Supplies), PKU 1 (Milupa). Some of these formulas are nutritionally complete and others require additional vitamins. In the older child a special amino-acid preparation such as Maxamaid XP (Scientific Hospital Supplies), Aminogran (Allen and Hanbury), and PKU 2 (Milupa) is used to provide the protein component of the diet. Some of these preparations contain vitamins and mineral, whereas others require supplements.

Phenylalanine is essential for growth and must not be eliminated completely from the diet. Once the initial high phenylalanine level is reduced with a phenylalanine-free diet, phenylalanine must be re-introduced by adding either breast milk or infant formula to the diet. In the case of the breast-fed baby, the phenylalanine-free infant formula is given in a measured quantity before the baby feeds from the breast. By monitoring the blood phenylalanine level regularly the amount of breast milk and therefore phenylalanine can be controlled by increasing or decreasing the measured phenylalanine-free formula. The larger the volume of phenylalanine-free formula the baby is given, the less breast milk he will take, and the smaller the volume the more he will take. The bottle-fed baby is given a known quantity of phenylalanine as measured infant formula (e.g. Cow & Gate Premium or SMA Gold Cap) and then allowed to feed freely on the phenylalanine-free formula.

In the older child the phenylalanine is supplied from measured portions of cereals and vegetable foods such as potato, rice, or breakfast cereals. The remaining energy requirements are met by including a variety of low-phenylalanine special products (flour, biscuits, pasta), fruits, and vegetables. Many of these special products are available on prescription to patients with phenylketonuria and constitute a very important part of the diet. Care should be taken not to confuse these products with gluten-free products which may contain large amount of protein and, therefore, phenylalanine.

In most centres, at the time of writing, a strict diet is recommended until the child is at least 10 years of age. After that time it may be possible to allow the blood phenylalanine levels to run within a higher range, thus enabling the diet to be less strict. The exact age at which the diet should be discontinued is not clear, if in fact it should be discontinued at all. There is a growing body of opinion that people with phenylketonuria should be on dietary restriction for life, although at present there is no evidence of either harm or benefit. There are important problems associated with a lifelong diet, particularly the cost of amino-acid supplements. It is our policy to maintain some degree of moderate protein restriction into adult life, using occasional blood phenylalanine levels as a yardstick. It is highly desirable that adults with phenylketonuria should continue to be seen from time to time, if only to ensure that relaxation of the diet is not causing them any harm. This poses some difficulty as it is not clear who should undertake this continued care. In some areas, paediatricians have established adult follow-up clinics.

A major new problem has arisen ironically as a result of the success in treating phenylketonuria. A generation of normal young women with phenylketonuria now exists. Their babies are at great risk of severe brain and other damage from high maternal phenylalanine levels. This damage occurs during a very early stage of embryonal development and may occur before the pregnancy is recognized. Phenylketonuric girls wishing to become pregnant must therefore follow a strict diet before conceiving and during pregnancy.

Phenylketonuria families can receive further information and support from National Society for Phenylketonuria and Allied Disorders. The Society also produces information to assist health professionals.

Galactosaemia

Galactose appears in the urine in three specific inborn errors of metabolism:

(1) classical galactosaemia;

(2) galactokinase deficiency;

(3) epimerase deficiency.

Classical galactosaemia

Galactosaemia is an autosomal recessive inherited disorder. The basic defect is a deficiency of galactose-1-phosphate uridyltransferase which is necessary to metabolize galactose to glucose phosphate. The incidence of classical galactosaemia is approximately 1:40 000 births.

The presentation depends on the severity of the disorder. Some infants die unexpectedly before the diagnosis is made. Less acute cases may have persisting neonatal jaundice with vomiting, diarrhoea, and impaired liver function with hepatomegaly. Some infants are referred because they are failing to thrive. Cataract may be present at an early stage.

Biochemical findings include a raised galactose-1-phosphate in erythrocytes. Initially the condition must be treated as a medical emergency because sudden death from hypoglycaemia is not unusual.

When a reducing substance other than glucose is found in the urine, the infant is started on a galactose-free diet immediately. This will lead to a rapid improvement and a reduction in the galactose-1-phosphate levels. The diet should be continued for life. With early diagnosis and strict dietary compliance one would expect a good outlook. Unfortunately, because some brain damage may have occurred prenatally, the long-term prognosis for intelligence is not as good as for phenylketonuria although many well-managed cases are of normal intelligence.

A galactose-free diet requires the exclusion of all galactose-containing foods. Galactose is a monosaccharide not generally found as such but as a component of the disaccharide lactose. It is therefore necessary to exclude all lactose from the diet, which in effect means following a milk-free diet. Care should also be taken to avoid other food and non-food items such as drugs and toothpaste which may contain lactose.

A soya formula such as Wysoy (Wyeth), Formula S (Cow & Gate), or a special preparation such as Galactomin 17 (Cow & Gate) should be used. It is no longer thought necessary to exclude galactosides because these do not affect galactose-1-phosphate levels. The diet therefore can include beans and pulses.

Children with galactosaemia should be followed regularly with monitoring of red blood cell galactose-1-phosphate levels and dietary review. It is important to arrange for psychological testing to be carried out from time to time.

Galactokinase deficiency

This disorder is due to a defect of the enzyme galactokinase and leads to accumulation of galactose in the ocular lens. It causes cataracts. Babies of mothers with the condition may be born with cataracts even though they do not have the disease.

Epimerase deficiency

This condition is similar to classical galactosaemia but is much more severe with a very poor prognosis.

Organic acidaemias

The term 'organic acidaemia' is applied to any condition in which there is elevation of an abnormal organic acid in the blood. Several of these rare disorders are caused by defects in the degradation of the essential branched-chain amino acids, leucine, valine, and isoleucine. The most common of these disorders are maple syrup urine disease, methylmalonic acidaemia, isovaleric acidaemia and proprionic acidaemia. The precise organic acid which is found varies with the site of the defect.

The more severe disorders in their classical form lead to ketosis, metabolic acidosis, vomiting, and neurological abnormalities in the newborn, with subsequent mental retardation if the child survives. Those less severely affected may present with recurring episodes of ketoacidosis, often precipitated by infections or a sudden increase in dietary protein and/or neurological problems, failure to thrive, or mental retardation.

The outcome for these children depends on several factors. Most important is whether the defect is due to a lack of the enzyme itself or whether it is due to a deficiency of the co-factor involved in the enzyme reaction. This in turn might be due to an abnormality in the utilization of the relevant vitamin. Such vitamin-dependent states are often highly responsive to mega doses of the vitamin involved. In some children where the defect is partial, the residual enzyme activity is relatively high, making control easier because the child can tolerate a less restrictive diet and may not become so acutely ill.

In vitamin-responsive disorders, if the diagnosis is made before irreversible damage and if treatment is begun sufficiently early, the outlook can be excellent. Even initially poorly-controlled cases may show a dramatic improvement in neurological function once the biochemical abnormality is under control. We have seen examples of children with apparently severe intellectual and psychomotor retardation as late as 10 months of age return to normal.

The dietary protein restriction required varies with the severity of the disorder. In some a special amino-acid supplement free from the offending branched-chain amino acid is necessary. The principles of the diet are similar to those used in phenylketonuria, but the exact dietary prescription must be tailored to the disorder and the individual child's requirements. In addition, parents should make regular checks for urinary ketones and report immediately if these increase. Regular measurement of blood and/or urine for the specific organic acid along with other biochemical monitoring should be performed.

The major difference from phenylketonuria is the potentially devastating consequences of not adhering to the diet, and the dramatic deterioration which can occur during a bout of inter-current infection or other illness. It is important to prevent the child becoming ketoacidotic and dehydrated. The parents are therefore advised to ensure that the child takes extra carbo-hydrates in the form of glucose, sugar, or glucose polymers during illness. It may be necessary to reduce the child's protein intake further, and extra fluids should be encouraged. If these measures do not induce a rapid improvement, the child should be admitted to hospital where an intravenous glucose drip may be required to prevent further ketoacidosis and dehydration, which if not checked can be fatal.

Because the child appears to be so well, parents can be lulled into a false sense of security. It is very important that they do not relax their vigilance or be tempted into thinking that the child is 'cured' and no longer at risk of an acute crisis.

RENAL DISEASE

General principles

Nutritional problems loom large in the management of children with chronic renal disease, particularly those who are in renal failure.

However, it is not only children with renal failure who need dietary help. There are many children with chronic renal con-ditions which will never cause renal failure or who will remain with relatively good renal function for many years. Some of these children have diseases which will eventually cause renal failure, whereas some conditions do not cause renal failure in themselves but may predispose to hypertension in later life. Good dietary care by an expert and experienced paediatric diet-itian is essential to the proper management of children with chronic renal disease, and is a principal reason why all such children with such diseases should attend a paediatric nephrology clinic.

Renal diseases not associated with renal failure

Risk of later hypertension

Any condition which damages or scars the renal parenchyma carries with it the risk that hypertension might subsequently develop. It is therefore particularly useful to offer healthy eating advice to children attending renal clinics. In essence this consists of the recommendations of the COMA panel on Diet and Cardiovascular Disease with emphasis placed on the need to avoid excess salt intake. Children who are overweight are offered help in reducing calorie intake.

Nephrotic syndrome

Most children with nephrotic syndrome have so called minimal change steroid-sensitive disease. It is thus usually possible to keep them free of proteinuria with its attendant risk of amino-acid deficiency and malnutrition. High-protein diets are not necessary. The main nutritional problem in these children is the obesity which may be associated with steroid therapy. Children vary enormously in the degree to which they become overweight with steroid treatment. The appetite is often enormously increased and in those with a predisposition to obesity quite alarming weight gain may ensue which in a few individuals does not revert on cessation of treatment. It may be wise if there is a family history of obesity to begin calorie restriction with the beginning of treatment rather than to wait until obesity has actually manifested itself.

In the approximately 5 per cent of childhood nephrotics who are steroid resistant, dietary management becomes relatively more important. Increased-protein, low-salt diets may help to reduce the oedema. Careful monitoring of the energy intake is desirable since many of these children have poor appetites.

Renal failure

Children with renal failure have major nutritional problems both during the period in which they are not in need of replacement renal therapy, i.e. dialysis and transplantation, and after the need for such management becomes imperative. As with other aspects of management, ideally diet and the changes it will undergo during different phases of the process should be seen by the child and its family as a logical progression, so that they will not be faced with sudden, unwelcome, and unpleasant dietary alterations.

It is essential to ensure that the parents and, in those old enough to understand, the child realize how important it is that the child should grow as near normally as possible and that this is linked to adequate intakes of nutrient and energy. For several reasons—some related to the underlying disease which cause the renal failure, some due to the effects of renal failure itself, and also because of important psychological factors —children with renal failure are often anorexic, eat poorly, and as a consequence suffer from malnutrition, and poor linear growth and weight gain. It is possible by ensuring that nutrition forms an integral part of management to obviate many of these difficulties.

Possibly the best way to consider the matter is to regard children with renal failure as typical as regards eating—only more so. In other words they are faddy, prone to cussedness when it comes to what they will eat or not eat, likely to use food as a weapon in the eternal battle with adults, and determined to want what is considered 'unhealthy' and to reject what is regarded as good. As with all children, the principle of success lies in gaining the confidence of the parents. In our experience, mothers who understand what is required and who are able to curb their natural anxiety are the ones whose children grow well. Poor growth is not an inevitable outcome of renal failure or long-term dialysis and some children with terminal renal failure grow close to their appropriate centiles.

The approach we use is to find out what the child finds acceptable and to attempt to build up energy and nutrient intake around this. The diet should be based on usual family eating patterns. If the household is one in which there is little food preparation or cooking, then it will be based on suitable processed foods, supplemented as necessary.

In our experience children with renal failure not yet requiring dialysis have a protein intake which tends to be quite low anyway. We have almost never resorted to severe restriction, because we believe that the theoretical benefits claimed by some are outweighed by the unpalatable diet and misery which is caused. Children on very restricted low-protein diets may stop growing because they drastically reduce their intake.

It is vitally important that the child has an adequate energy intake. Using information based on dietary assessment, energy intake is supplemented by using normal foods and special dietary products. In some children, sodium and potassium restriction is required. The dietary prescription will vary greatly during the course of renal failure and in individual children.

Once the child is on renal replacement therapy, the diet is tailored to the type of treatment and to the individual child's requirements. For example, on peritoneal dialysis, a high-protein diet is necessary, whereas on haemodialysis, a lower protein intake is appropriate.

Vitamin supplementation is desirable for all children with renal failure because of the reduced intake of normal foods. This is best given as a standard multi-vitamin preparation. In addition it is our policy to give vitamin D either as calcitriol or alpha-calcidol once the blood creatinine is clearly elevated. Although this requires careful monitoring of the blood calcium initially, it avoids the possibility of metabolic bone disease.

Monitoring of growth

The best index of success is growth and therefore it is essential that a good record be kept of height and weight measurements, which should be plotted on a centile chart. While many children with renal failure or other chronic renal disease grow quite well until before puberty, they often have delay in the pubertal growth spurt which may not be due to dietary or metabolic factors. Such children will sometimes show surprising catch-up during mid-adolescence.

DIABETES MELLITUS

Diabetes mellitus in children invariably takes the form of juvenile diabetes mellitus which requires insulin. Symptoms cannot usually be treated using tablets as with some forms of maturity onset diabetes mellitus. The classical symptoms of juvenile diabetes mellitus are an acute onset with polyuria, polydipsia, weight loss, raised blood sugar, and glycosuria. The treatment of insulin injections and diet aim to normalize blood glucose levels, enabling the child to lead a fully active normal life.

The child should be referred immediately to the local paediatric diabetic team so that treatment can be commenced. In most areas the child will be admitted to hospital for one to two weeks. However, in some areas a diabetic home-care team has been developed and the diabetic child can be stabilized at home. The aim of initial treatment is to normalize the blood glucose level by giving appropriate insulin injections along with a suitable diet. During this time the child and family are taught the basics of treatment. This includes testing blood or urine glucose, insulin injections, recognition of different insulins, drawing up the correct dose, injection technique, rotation of injection sites, and care of syringe and needles. They are also taught the basic principles of the diet, and what they should do in an emergency.

Further teaching includes dealing with hypoglycaemia, the possible need for extra carbohydrate during exercise, going on holiday, and other problems of daily life as they occur. These and other refinements of treatment can be learned over a longer period of time.

The dietary treatment for the diabetic child aims to provide a nutritionally balanced diet, incorporating healthy eating practices and adequate nutrition for optimal growth. When the child is first seen by the dietitian a dietary history will be taken and the dietary prescription made using the assessment and taking into account the child's nutritional requirements. This can be achieved by eating a diet high in fibre, low in fat, with between 45 per cent and 55 per cent of the energy provided by carbohydrate. Adequate energy is essential and the requirements will vary according to the age, size, and activity of the child. If the diet is inadequate the child will be perpetually hungry. The diet is normally based on a carbohydrate exchange system and the children are advised to divide the daily carbohydrate allowance between three meals and three snacks.

A quick method for calculating the carbohydrate requirement is 100 g of carbohydrate plus 10 g for every year of life. Thus a six-year-old child will take 160 g. This method can be used to provide a temporary prescription, but each individual child's carbohydrate requirements are different and the diet must, therefore, in the long term be based on the dietitians assessment. The carbohydrate should be divided between three meals and three snacks according to the child's usual meal pattern and the type of insulin. This initial carbohydrate prescription usually requires modification within the first few weeks, often after the child has regained any weight lost.

The carbohydrates are divided into 10 g exchanges. One carbohydrate exchange when eaten in a specified amount contains 10 g of carbohydrate (Table 10.2). The British Diabetic Association produces a list of standard carbohydrate exchanges and information regarding the carbohydrate content of manufactured foods (Countdown).

Families with a diabetic child are advised to join the British Diabetic Association and children are encouraged to participate

Table 10.2. Examples of 10-g carbohydrate exchanges

Food	Household measure	Weight
Wholemeal bread	small slice	25g
White bread	small thin slice	17g
Rice crispies	6 tablespoons	10g
Weetabix	1 biscuit	15g
Plain semi-sweet biscuit	2 biscuits	15g
Digestive biscuit	1 biscuit	15g
Boiled potato	1 egg sized	50g
Chips	4–5 average	25g
Apple	1 medium	110g
Orange	1 large	150g
Orange juice (unsweetened)	7 tablespoons	100g
Whole milk	1/3 pint	200ml

in the diabetic camps organized by the association. The camps are supervised by trained staff including doctors, nurses, and dietitians, and provide the diabetic child with the chance to meet others with the same condition and to learn how they cope with their diabetes. The children are encouraged to participate in a wide range of activities and are taught about self care and control of their condition.

MAJOR GASTRO-INTESTINAL DISEASES

This section briefly discusses some of the major gastro-intestinal diseases which effect children, other than acute diarrhoea and gastroenteritis which are dealt with in earlier chapters. If any of the following conditions are suspected, the child should be referred to a specialist centre where the diagnosis can be confirmed and appropriate treatment commenced.

Severe chronic intractable diarrhoea in infancy

Very rarely an episode of what appears to be simple gastroenteritis in an infant fails to resolve and continues unrelentingly with dehydration, electrolyte disturbance, and progressive malnutrition. Investigations usually fail to reveal an explanation for the problem. The outlook for such children is often poor and careful evaluation in a centre for paediatric gastro-enterology may be appropriate.

Maintaining nutrition in such cases can become a nigh impossible task. Even the most elemental of feeds may not be tolerated and special preparations such a Comminuted Chicken Meat (Cow & Gate) may be tried. Total parenteral nutrition may be required but there is evidence that the prognosis is not improved by this. Some experts have suggested that fresh human milk may help some of these babies.

Inflammatory bowel disease

This term describes two conditions which occur in childhood, ulcerative colitis and Crohn's disease. Although clinically similar in some ways, the treatment and long-term outlook are quite different.

Crohn's disease

Crohn's disease is a chronic inflammatory disorder that may affect any part of the alimentary tract with a characteristic pattern of clinical and pathological features. Clinical features include abdominal pain, which may be the dominant symptom, fever, diarrhoea, growth reduction, anorexia, and anaemia. Some children present with mouth ulcers or anal fissures. There is some evidence that this condition is becoming more common.

The disease follows a very irregular relapsing course and it can be very difficult to be sure whether treatment is effective. It is an intractable disease which may continue for years. The long-term outlook for childhood cases is not clear.

Remission of symptoms can be achieved with drugs such as sulphasalazine. In children with chronic involvement, short-term corticosteroid therapy and/or immunosuppressive therapy with azathioprine have been found to be very useful.

One of the major problems is to maintain normal growth in these children, and nutritional support is an important part of treatment. Dietary treatments of different types may be used, varying from simple nutritional supplementation to provide a high-protein, high-energy diet, to exclusion and elemental diets. Some recent work has shown that the use of elemental diets can induce and maintain remission. Some authorities have advocated exclusion diets and this may be worth trying in resistant cases. Total parenteral nutrition can also induce remission.

Surgery is usually reserved for patients with complications such as obstruction, toxic megacolon, fistulae, and abscesses, and those whose symptoms do not respond to medical treatment. It is sometimes advocated to achieve a remission just before the expected pubertal growth spurt to avoid permanent stunting of growth, particularly in those children who have had much steroid therapy.

Ulcerative colitis

Ulcerative colitis usually presents with diarrhoea with or without bleeding, but in some cases may follow a rapidly progressive course with acute toxic megacolon which requires urgent surgery. Extra-intestinal complications include iritis, arthritis, and liver damage. It follows an unpredictable relapsing course and undernutrition is an important sequel.

The dietary treatment for ulcerative colitis is usually to ensure that the child has an adequate nutritional intake with a high protein, high energy intake. The majority of children with ulcerative colitis will eventually have to undergo colectomy because of the risk of colonic cancer in later life, but unlike Crohn's disease the operation is curative.

FURTHER READING AND REFERENCES

Berenson, G. S. (1986). *Cardiovascular risk factors in children*. Raven Press, New York.

British National Formulary (1988). British Medical Association and The Pharmaceutical Society of Great Britain.

Craig, O. (1982). *Childhood diabetes—the facts*. Oxford University Press, Oxford.

Department of Health and Social Security (1980). *Artificial feeds for the young infant*. HMSO, London.

Department of Health and Social Security (1987). *Diet and cardiovascular disease (COMA)*. HMSO, London.

Department of Health and Social Security (1987). *Present day practice in infant feeding*. HMSO, London.

Department of Health and Social Security (1989). *The diets of British school children*. HMSO, London.

Francis, D. (1987). *Diets for sick children*. Blackwell Scientific Publications, Oxford.

Francis, D. (1987). *Nutrition for children*. Blackwell Scientific Publications, Oxford.

Martin, J. and White, A. (1988). *Infant feeding 1985*. HMSO, London.

McCance, R. and Widdowson, E. (1978). *The composition of food*. HMSO, London.

McLaren D. S. and Burman, D. (1989). *Textbook of Paediatric Nutrition*. Churchill Livingstone, New York.

Rawcliffe, P. and Rolf, R. (1985). *The gluten-free diet book*. Dunitz.

Royal College of Midwives (1988). *Successful breastfeeding—A practical guide for midwives*. Holywell Press, Oxford.

Taitz, L. S. (1983). *The obese child*. Blackwell Scientific Press, Oxford.

Thomas, B. (1987). *Manual of dietetic practice*. Blackwell Scientific Publications, Oxford.

Wharton, B. A. (ed.) (1982). Food for the suckling. *Acta Paediatrica Scandinavica* (Suppl. 299).

Wharton, B. A. (ed.) (1986). Food for the weanling. Conference on feeding the older infant and toddler. *Acta Paediatrica Scandinavica* (Suppl. 323).

Wharton, B. A. (ed.) (1987). Symposium on child nutrition. *Nutrition and Health*.

Wharton, B. A. (1987). *Nutrition and feeding of preterm infants.* Blackwell Scientific Publications, Oxford.

Walker-Smith, J. (1987). *Practical paediatric gastroenterology.* Butterworths, London.

Workman, E. Hunter, J., and Alun Jones, V. (1984). *The allergy diet.* Dunitz.

Further nutrition and dietetic information can be obtained from:

1. Your local hospital dietetic department.
2. The British Dietetic Association,
   Daimler House, Paradise Circus, Queensway,
   Birmingham B1 2BJ.

SELF-HELP GROUPS

Anorexic Aid
The Priory Centre, 11 Priory Road, High Wycombe, Bucks.

Anorexic Family Aid
Sackville Place, 44 Magdelen Street, Norwich, Norfolk NR3 1JE.

Association of Breast Feeding Mothers
131 Mayow Road, London SE26 4HZ.

British Diabetic Association
10 Queen Anne Street, London W1M 0BD.

The British Kidney Patient Association
BUPA, Bordon, Hants.

The Coeliac Society of the United Kingdom
P.O. Box 220, High Wycombe, Bucks. HP11 2HY.

Cystic Fibrosis Research Trust
Alexandra House, 5 Blyth Road, Bromley, Kent BR1 3RS.

Down's Children's Association
4 Oxford Street, London W1N 0FL.

Family Heart Association (The Familial Hypercholesterolaemia and Familial Hyperlipidaemia Association)
P.O. Box 116, Kidlington, Oxford OX5 1DT.

Foresight (Association for Promotion of Pre-conceptual Care)
c/o Mrs Barnes, The Old Vicarage, Church Lane, Whitley, Godalming, Surrey GU8 SPN.

Hyperactive Children's Support Group
59 Meadowside, Angmering, Sussex BN16 4BW.

La Leche League of Great Britain
BM 3424 London WC1 6XX.

The Migraine Trust
45 Great Ormond Street, London W2 3TB.

The National Childbirth Trust
9 Queensborough Terrace, London W2 3TB.

National Eczema Society
Tavistock House, North Tavistock Square, London WC1H 9SR.

National Federation of Kidney Patients' Associations
'Acorn Lodge', Woodsetts, Nr Worksop, Notts. S81 8AT.

The National Society for Phenylketonuria and Allied Disorders Limited
26 Towngate Grove, Mirfield, West Yorkshire.

Prader Willi Syndrome Association (UK)
30 Follet Drive, Abbots Langley, Herts. WD5 0LP.

The Research Trust for Metabolic Diseases in Children
9 Arnold Street, Nantwich, Cheshire CW5 5QB.

The Spastics Society
12 Park Crescent, London W1N 4EQ.

INDEX